The Accidental Caregiver

THE ACCIDENTAL CAREGIVER

Wisdom and Guidance for the Unexpected Challenges of Family Caregiving

KIMBERLY FRASER

sh.
SUTHERLAND
HOUSE
TORONTO, 2022

Sutherland House
416 Moore Ave., Suite 205
Toronto, ON M4G 1C9

First edition, October 2022

If you are interested in inviting one of our authors to a live event or media appearance, please contact sranasinghe@sutherlandhousebooks.com and visit our website at sutherlandhousebooks.com for more information about our authors and their schedules.

We acknowledge the support of the Government of Canada.

Manufactured in Turkey
Cover designed by Lena Yang

Library and Archives Canada Cataloguing in Publication
Title: The accidental caregiver : wisdom and guidance for the unexpected challenges of family caregiving / Kimberly Fraser.
Names: Fraser, Kimberly, author.
Identifiers: Canadiana 20220234396 | ISBN 9781989555811 (softcover)
Subjects: LCSH: Caregivers.
Classification: LCC RA645.3 .F73 2022 | DDC 649.8—dc23

ISBN 978-1-989555-81-1

To my parents

To my father, Donald Polley. Dad, you have always been my North Star in life, in sickness, and in death.

To my mother, Myrna Polley. Mom you are my inspiration. The love and care you gave not only to Dad, but to all of us over the years is immeasurable. You are the consummate caregiver.

CONTENTS

Foreword   xi

Introduction: How It Began   1

Chapter 1: A New Normal   7

Chapter 2: Resilience   18

Chapter 3: Change, Loss, and Grief   35

Chapter 4: Home Care and Other Services   63

Chapter 5: Respite   99

Chapter 6: Information Needs   111

Chapter 7: Beat the Clock   140

Chapter 8: Meaningful Conversations   150

Chapter 9: A Sense of Self   179

Chapter 10: Mapping Your Way   196

Afterword   206

Gratitude   219

Glossary   223

FOREWORD

THIS IS A BOOK FOR everyone.

Most of us have been caregivers, are currently caregivers, or will one day become caregivers. Many of us will eventually need caregivers. Some of us are professionals who care for those who are ill but can provide exemplary care only if we understand the experiences and challenges of their caregivers.

This book is necessary as there aren't many tools or practical handbooks available to caregivers. Caregivers need this book because, as the title suggests, they assume the caregiving role unexpectedly, and usually without the training or knowledge to handle the diverse tasks and stresses they will have to manage. Even the author herself, a nurse with a background directing a large home support business, in a family of nurses, found it a struggle when her father needed increasing levels of care.

Before becoming caregivers, many might have said that they couldn't manage such ongoing, complex responsibility for another person; and yet most find themselves able and ready when the time comes, mustering the inner strength to get on with it. In addition to providing personal care, caregivers assume a leading role in researching illness and best approaches to management, treatment options, and access to resources. They may also be powerful advocates, not only for their loved ones but for a better and more responsive health care system.

Dr. Kimberly Fraser is an ideal person to shine a light on the humanity, the sense of loss and life change, the demands, the rewards, the support needs, and the personal costs of caregiving. She has extensive personal as well as professional experience: her father, who I knew, had progressive MS, and she writes about the challenges this presented to her mother and herself with frank honesty.

As a neurologist whose research unit cared for patients with MS, I needed to understand the abilities, challenges, resources, and coping skills of our patients' caregivers. Since there was no literature to guide us when we began in the 1970s, we did some of our own research. At that point, all of the published studies focused on women as care-givers and appeared in nursing journals; yet in the case of MS, 75% of the caregivers were men. We were interested in how they fared in this role. Our research unit found, despite a popular prejudice, that men were good caregivers, although there were some differences. They took caregiving on more like a project, whereas female caregivers adopted the role as a natural process. We also found the male caregivers were better at taking care of their own health than women, but were more reluctant to seek support, especially from outside agencies, as they tended to feel this meant they were failing as caregivers. Overall, the care they provided was impressive, perhaps because they usually had a long time to ease into the role. But this book would have been a great help for both patients and caregivers to allow them to plan and prepare. It also would have helped us to better focus on many of the issues so clearly voiced by our patients.

I learned more when my family and I became caregivers for my mother-in-law, who battled dementia, and later my daughter, who died of a brain tumor. Although I have been a physician for half a century, my career caring for MS patients did not prepare me for the role of caregiver. I had to learn along with my wife and four children, who rose to the challenge with love and skill as we dealt with each day as it came. Everyone had busy lives and family responsibilities but adjusted to help, even when this required adopting a shared rotating twenty-four-hour schedule.

The structure of this book presents a series of central issues in caregiving, powerfully underlined by interviews and personal stories. The voices of the caregivers are clear, even eloquent. Their stories are sometimes difficult to hear, but all are instructive. Dr. Fraser has interviewed seventy-five caregivers, and of course has interacted with hundreds of others over the course of her career.

Part of her innovative approach has been to organize creative workshops using collage in which caregivers were encouraged to identify words and images that captured the essence of their caregiving experience. The arts clearly can do a lot to help patients to cope with, understand, and learn from their experiences. Expressive art, collage making, and journaling are all examples of creative enterprises that can be of significant benefit to caregivers and patients alike.

In these workshops, many of the caregivers Dr. Fraser interviews describe feeling like prisoners due to inadequate support, constant demands, and a sense of being cut off from friends, community, and their normal social lives. They lose the loved one they once knew, even though that person is still physically present. One woman speaks of being a widow with a husband. There is also a loss of sense of self as normal life fades into the caregiving process.

The voices of the caregivers featured here remind me that our approach to health care often has a missing element. We have been admonished in recent times to remember the individual when we are diagnosing and treating illness. Sir William Osler, the famed Canadian physician of the nineteenth century, said, "Ask not what disease the person has, but rather what person the disease has." That is wise, but it ignores the other person in the room who also requires information, resources, and support, and who is also suffering. They, too, have needs—and attention paid to them will be reflected in better care for the patient.

The Covid-19 pandemic brought to light the importance of caregiving in our society. The devotion and hard work of families is often invisible when health care is considered as a purely institutional and administrative system. During the pandemic, family members could not enter care facilities where they had often complemented the care provided by professionals and staff, contributed important emotional and social support, and enhanced the quality of life of the patients. Although the role of families rarely makes it to a flow sheet or budget consideration, the crisis reminded everyone of the vital role of families in health care.

We are way behind, despite the fact that demographers have been warning us for decades of the growing numbers of people who will require care as boomers age. The number of families involved in caregiving will continually grow, and we will need to grow the funding, resources, innovations, and assistance to support them.

This book is a valuable resource for everyone. In it, caregivers and patients will find helpful insights to process the challenges they are negotiating; family and friends will learn about ways they can be supportive; legislators will notice the deficiencies in this important aspect of our health care system; and health professionals will be reminded that attention to caregivers is crucial to providing the best care for their patients.

* * *

Dr. T. Jock Murray, OC, ONS, MD, FRCPC, MACP, FAAN, FRCP, FCAHS, is Professor Emeritus and former Dean of Medicine at Dalhousie University. He has received many awards for contributions to MS, medical education, medical humanities, and medical history, and has been awarded five honorary degrees, the Order of Canada, and the Order of Nova Scotia. He has been inducted into the Canadian Medical Hall of Fame and the Discovery Center Hall of Fame.

INTRODUCTION

How It Began

ONCE YOU KNOW SOMETHING, YOU can't unknow it. The lives of family caregivers and their stories have been a part of me for more than thirty-five years. They have propelled me forward in my nursing, my research, my policy advocacy, and now in my writing.

When people find out what I do for a living, they tell me stories that demonstrate the spectrum of emotions that are inherent in family caregiving. I hear stories about caregivers feeling gratitude that they can actually devote the time and energy to the role and how they would never want anyone else to do what they are doing for their loved one. But conversely, and perhaps more often, I hear stories that break my heart. That's the feeling I had when a family caregiver, Carol, told me how she felt one New Year's Day. When other people were feeling the rise of enthusiasm that new beginnings can bring, she said, "I woke up and thought to myself, *oh here we go, year three of an indefinite sentence.*" Every time family caregivers shared some version of their life, I made a promise to myself that I would find ways to pass along their stories. This book is one of those ways.

Reading about the challenges others have faced can support us in our own struggles. We gain insight by seeing how they handle situations similar to our own. Yet as much as we recognize ourselves in stories as more than numbers, we can't ignore the current caregiving crisis in North America, nor can we overlook the fact that the demographic shift caused by aging boomers means that this crisis is only going to grow. With an increasing number of older persons comes an increasing number of people requiring care. Add to that the declining birth rate and insufficient health human resources—nurses, doctors, and other health care providers—and many of us will be looking after not just one person in our lifetime, but multiple people. We will care for a parent or an in-law, sibling or other relative, and even neighbors or friends in our lifetime. As former first lady Rosalynn Carter says, "There are only four kinds of people in the world: those who have been caregivers, those who are currently caregivers, those who will be caregivers, and those who will need caregivers." Without a doubt, we are ill-prepared.

Currently, there are about 8 million Canadians, or 28% of the population fifteen years and over, providing care to family members with a long-term health problem, disability, or problems related to aging and frailty. It is estimated that 46% of people over fifteen years of age will be a caregiver at some point in their life. Some will even care for two or three people over the course of their lifetime. In the United States, an estimated 65 million Americans provided unpaid care to someone in 2016, up from the 43.5 million who reported caring for someone the prior year. The statistics are sobering.

Who is a Caregiver?

One in four Canadians (7.8 million) are family caregivers. Almost half (47%) are caring for a parent or parent-in-law, 13% are caring for their spouse or partner, and 8% for their child with a long-term medical condition or disability. The remaining provide care to a close friend or neighbor (13%), or other extended family member (19%). The numbers are proportionately similar in the United States, Australia, the United Kingdom, and other European nations.

Despite being more than 65 million strong, the American population of family caregivers is often viewed as a homogenous group. However, this is no more the case in the United States than elsewhere in the developed world. Policy-makers and program coordinators tend to overlook the crucial differences between people who are taking care of an ill spouse and those who are looking after an aging parent.

The typical caregiver is between forty and seventy years old, with spousal caregivers being slightly older—between sixty and eighty years old. Given the growing number of young people in caregiving roles, their unique needs cannot be overlooked. It is society's obligation to provide better care and support to caregivers who are providing tremendous economic benefits to their countries. Caregivers contribute an estimated 31 billion dollars annually in Canada, 470 billion in the United States, and 200 billion in the United Kingdom. These figures are not insignificant.

The Essence of Intimate Family Caregiving

The characters and stories in this book introduce the reader to real-life accounts of family caregivers I encountered through my work in home care nursing, my research on family caregiving, and witnessing my mother care for my father for twenty-one years. I write about intimate family caregivers in personal relationships with the individual they are caring for. They may be spouses, mothers, fathers, daughters, sons, nieces, nephews, siblings, or close friends. They are unpaid individuals who provide care and support to loved ones; most often, but not always, they live with the person they are caring for. Intimate family caregivers rarely choose this role, but they take it on with strength, resilience, and creativity as they learn to live according to a new normal.

By sharing these sometimes-difficult experiences, I hope that not only will you feel less alone but you will also see the joy and optimism displayed by many. Over the course of the next ten chapters, I will demonstrate the ways in which caregivers adapt to their "new normal" with resilience in the face of constant change, grief, and loss. Caregivers sometimes don't know what they don't know. I will talk about how to find information that can lead to better supports and services, including home care and obtaining respite care that works. I will share ways caregivers manage their time—something always in short supply. Talking with caregivers and offering support to them is not always easy, so I will offer ways to have meaningful conversations both as a caregiver and with a caregiver. While every caregiving journey has a different trajectory, there are similarities in the twists and turns as caregivers navigate their course, find ways to carve out time for their own needs, and learn to maintain a sense of self.

There are encouraging moments involved in caregiving and positive effects to be derived. This book includes creative solutions and effective coping strategies shared by caregivers who believed that, in spite of everything, they were the best person to care for their loved one. These solutions and strategies are effective whether you care for someone in your home, in their home, or in a facility like a long-term care center. Family caregiving crosses all boundaries and will affect all of us at some point in our lives.

My Story

My father was diagnosed with primary progressive multiple sclerosis (MS) when he was forty-three and in the prime of his life. A proud husband and father of four, he was strong and active, and highly engaged in community life. My mother was a registered nurse who became Dad's primary caregiver for twenty-one years until he died at home. When my maternal grandmother was in her early seventies, she moved next door. In the later years of Nanna's life, and at a time when Dad's disease had advanced to a stage where he needed full-time care, Mom became a dual caregiver. Her story, our family's story, is woven through the pages of this book along with the stories of nine other families I have come to know, mostly through my research.

As I grew into my nursing career, I gravitated to settings where family nursing was embodied—the community, and particularly home care. I can't say it was planned, but each step brought me closer to family caregivers and their experiences with the health care system. Over the years I saw all kinds of family/friend caregiver relationships. Some resembled my family's experience, others did not. Some had a lot of support, both formally from the health care system and from other family members. But many did not get what that they needed or expected, either from those close to them or from Canada's supposedly world-class health care system. What an eye-opener that was.

I began my career as a frontline community health nurse and soon entered leadership roles. I was a nursing educator prior to becoming a nurse entrepreneur and administrator for nearly twenty-five years, developing a large home health care company and a licensed private vocational school to educate health care aides. During those years I was curious about how we make some of the decisions we make in health care—at all policy and practice levels—so I went back to school for my PhD. In the last fifteen years I have been a nurse researcher and professor, with an interest in and focus on home care and family caregiving.

I am passionate about the plight of the family caregiver. It is a future that concerns me. The contribution of family caregivers in Canada, the United States, and most developed countries is well documented by governments and NGOs alike. It is an undisputable fact that family caregivers are bearing the burden of caring for loved ones who need assistance with physical, mental, or developmental limitations, as well as an aging population, many of whom are living with multiple chronic conditions. Yet, unless someone has first-hand knowledge about family caregiving (either through taking on the responsibility themselves or witnessing up-close and personal another family member in the role), they cannot be aware of what is involved, nor can they appreciate the sacrifices and rewards. My intention is to tell true accounts about what I have learned through the course of my career, and as a daughter of a family caregiver.

Having interviewed over seventy-five family caregivers, and listened to countless others who have shared their stories with me, I hope to bring awareness to the issue and spark a broader and deeper dialogue among concerned people. Because only by opening up what goes on behind closed doors will we begin to gain traction and mobilize the necessary change to better support caregivers.[1]

---

[1] All of the stories in this book are completely factual; certain identifying details have been altered to protect the privacy of some people.

CHAPTER ONE

A New Normal

"The stress level is high. I'm sad, I'm overwhelmed, I'm frustrated. This is my one joy" (she points to her dog).

—Jeanette

My Mother and Father

MY EARLIEST EXPOSURE TO FAMILY caregiving was personal. In December 1980, during my first term at nursing school, my father was diagnosed with primary progressive MS. Dad was forty-three and Mom was forty-one. Their lives changed forever. *Our* lives changed forever.

Far less was known about primary progressive MS at the time, and fewer drugs and interventions were available for symptom management. The condition becomes debilitating over time, but the speed and severity of the disease is different in everybody. About seven years after my Dad's diagnosis, my mother became his caregiver.

Dad went quickly from his full-time work as a manager at the Nova Scotia Department of Mines and Energy to part-time, until he was fully retired on a disability pension at forty-six. He stayed involved with his community service work, reading his mail, and watching stocks and bonds. He even took his stockbroker course but couldn't write the test because his mind wasn't as sharp (he wasn't confused, just not fully able to process details). A Shriner and a Mason, Dad was able to attend the various lodge meetings only with the help of family and friends. It wasn't always easy or without incident—there were falls and stumbles—and over time, he progressed from crutches to a wheelchair. Being in the wheelchair affected his social and community life, and with his general deterioration came fatigue and decreased muscle tone. When his speech was affected, he found it increasingly difficult to hold his head upright without support. Ultimately, he let go of his participation in lodge and church. It was a sad and significant marker of the effect the disease was having on his life.

Mom had to retire from her nursing position when it was no longer safe for Dad to be alone for long periods. This was about ten years after his diagnosis and much sooner than she had planned, but it was becoming impossible for her to cope with the competing demands of work and home. When on day shifts at the hospital, she'd get Dad up and settled in his chair before leaving at 6:30 AM. After her twelve-hour shift ended at 7:00 PM, Mom would rush home to see to him. By then, only one of my siblings, Tara, was living at home, working while she attended nursing school. (Yes, we were a family of nurses.) When Mom was on nights, she'd get home at 7:30 AM, at which time Dad was ready to get out of bed. She'd cook his breakfast, help him wash and dress, and get him into his wheelchair so he could go to the den, our family room, for the day. Mom would get him sitting comfortably in his reclining chair with everything he needed nearby, all before she went to bed at 9:30 AM.

Some days Dad would call out to her if he spilt his urinal or fell out of his chair reaching for something. It was a worrisome time for Mom. She felt tremendous stress in her body due to the constant rush to get things done. Her blood pressure went up and she required medication. She often experienced stomach upset and sheer exhaustion.

Mom and Dad had a solid marriage. They respected each other and showed love and affection openly. They also had no problem saying when they were upset about something, though it was rarely directed at the other. My mother was a strong woman, but the life she had enjoyed during the first twenty years of marriage was long gone. Mom was pragmatic. "It's hard," she often said. "It's not the life we imagined. He's not the husband I married." Their life changed dramatically as a new reality set in. She worked as a nurse as long as was feasible. She obtained whatever care and equipment Dad needed, learned new skills, and advocated for Dad—a lot. Mom was pragmatic. A doer. And she faced caregiving head on. There was no alternative.

We still don't know enough about MS. This disease of the central nervous system, which disrupts the flow of information within the brain, and between the brain and the body, is unpredictable. Exacerbating remitting MS, which is the most common form of the disease, is characterized by attacks, followed by periods of partial or complete remission in which symptoms may disappear. Exacerbating remitting MS may develop into primary progressive MS, but it may not. Unfortunately, Dad had primary progressive MS, and his health deteriorated rapidly.

My father was never confused, but he did become a bit dull in his affect. He couldn't think or process information as fast as he used to. He grew to rely on clichés, which drove Mom nuts. I remember walking into the den on one of my visits home. Dad was sitting in his dark blue recliner rocker, next to a steel pole my brother had drilled into the floor and the ceiling. Dad hung onto it as he maneuvered from his wheelchair to his recliner and used it to pull himself up if he needed to reach something or take pressure off his back and bottom as he changed positions.

I swung myself around his pole as I reached down to give him a hug and a kiss. "Hi, Dad, what's new? How are you?"

"Oh, you know, dear, the same. They treat me like a mushroom around here. They keep me in the dark and feed me a bunch of shit." He chuckled, proud of his wit.

His grey stubble was obvious. Now that he was shaving with his electric razor, he never got the smooth finish he used to. I reached for his ear and pulled it forward to have a look. This had become routine, because one of his caregivers always slathered on the lotion but rarely scrubbed behind his ears well enough. This meant it often built up, congealed, and hardened—almost like the rind over a rich old cheese. It angered me so much, the way she'd give him such a quick wash without paying much attention. So, I helped him when I was home. "I'm getting a face cloth and scrubbing behind your ears again, Dad. I can't stand that. It must feel gross!"

"No matter, dear."

I left the den to fetch a face cloth. As I walked back through the kitchen, I stopped to hug Mom. Her brown eyes rolled as she shook her head. "I heard your father and those damn clichés! He just can't help himself." She paused before continuing. "My God, I get tired of listening to them. Clarence was down the other day and you know that silly bastard, leaping around the room talking stocks. Donnie can't talk about that stuff anymore. Clarence goes on and your father repeats the same old, same old. He either says that he's *just like a mushroom, call a spade a spade,* or *you seen one you seen 'em all.*"

She took a deep breath and laughed. "Goodness," she said. "I'm going to dive off the deep end."

"Mom, I don't know how to tell you this, but 'dive off the deep end' is a cliché." We both cracked up at that.

The Physical and Emotional Toll

I'll never forget the day of Mom's big confession. It was about seven years after Dad's diagnosis, around the time she retired to take care of him full-time. "What you kids and everybody else see on the outside is not what I really feel," she told me. "Inside, I'm a *seething bitch*." That she said it with such conviction was what shocked me. I didn't have a clue how to respond.

My mother could be quite funny, or at least she used to be. She was smart, compassionate, and to me, the consummate caregiver. Always sharp witted and honest, she told me she couldn't fully embrace the bitch thing or *she* might be gone forever. I knew what she meant. Dad's diagnosis had ripped the life my parents had planned right out from under them. How could she not feel anger and resentment? And yet, she believed that if she let that bitterness take over, she wouldn't be able to go on and live the life they had now—the new normal.

Mom gave over her life to care for Dad and meet his every need. Sometimes she'd get frustrated. My parents used to talk a lot right up until the time my father could no longer carry on a conversation, which happened about three years before he died.

"What are you baking out there?" he would ask if he heard the beaters going.

"Oh, just a Boston crème pie. All of a sudden I had a hankering for that and I remembered I had a frozen pie crust in the freezer so I'm just making the filling and the icing for it."

"That'll be good, dear. Bob Barker is coming on right away."

"I'll be right in as soon as I get this in the oven and finish peeling the potatoes for supper."

My parents still found joy in some of the old habits, like watching their favorite TV shows and eating their favorite meals. Many people take comfort in the familiar. Indeed, that's a big part of learning how to cope: understanding that, while so many things have changed, not everything has. This is true as much for relationships as it is for routines.

Dad was never demanding. Thankfully, he never became nasty or difficult, or had personality changes, traits that sometimes affect people with MS. For that, I often said a prayer of thanks.

My father loved and appreciated everything Mom ever did for him, no matter how big or small. And she was never angry at Dad, just at the tragic, horrid circumstances caused by a chronic, life-limiting illness. Mom was mad as hell that her handsome, strong, capable husband got one of the nastiest, most debilitating, and often family-destroying diseases of the twentieth century. There was no cure, and for Dad there was little treatment. It was unbelievable to us kids that our family future was no longer what we'd had in mind. Dad's life was taken from him and Mom's from her. Dad comes from a family of long-lived people, and MS doesn't kill you in and of itself (the patient usually dies of some other cause or complication, rather than the disease). So, Mom knew she was in for a life sentence.

Caregiving exacts a toll that is emotional as well as physical. Mom was pissed off at the world, with a lot of love sprinkled in. Through the twenty-one years of caregiving for Dad, there was laughter, weddings, babies, health crises, bad health care, tons of advocacy, and discussions with crazy decision-makers and health care administrators. There were wonderful caregivers and some who didn't seem to care. There were system obstacles—lots of them—to overcome, as well as love. Without love, I'm not sure what would have happened to us. We were in it for the long haul. There was no escape. It was exhausting, frustrating, and burdensome. But it was what it was.

The flip side of all the sadness, burden, and frustration is that most caregivers wouldn't give up their role for any reason. Citing love and a compulsion to care for their loved one, they say "If not me, then who?" Caregivers want to give, to help, *to be there.* Good thing too, because the role is all-consuming—physically, spiritually, and emotionally. It is unreal. It is real. It is pain and suffering, love and courage. It is also life in its every breath.

Understanding Caregiving: A Creative Approach

Several years ago, I led an arts-based research study on home care and family caregiving. I was passionate about the cause, as I have long believed that a creative approach will help people uncover far more than interviews and dialogue alone. I learned early in my career that if I asked someone about a particular experience—how they felt when the home care nurse came or what it was like to see their loved one decline—I would often be met by vague and generic answers. "Oh," they'd say. "Well, it was difficult, I guess. Seeing Mom like that." However, if they were involved in creating something such as a collage, a poem, or even a doodle, their responses would become deeper, more reflective. Creativity helps the brain remember more clearly. Looking at pictures or photos can have a similar effect, in that it causes us to switch from using our analytical left brain to our intuitive right brain, which engages our emotions.

Art is a powerful medium that encourages deeper reflections and insights. It can cause us to look at things differently, which in turn can lead to positive change, such as seeking a therapist, or asking for more support from home care, family members, or physicians. Some caregivers saw that they needed a break, so they enlisted the help of their children. One man looked into a day program so his wife could get out of the home a few days each week. Sure, sometimes nothing can be done to alter a situation, but even this realization can help people view their circumstances through a different lens. That in itself can encourage a new approach to self-care so that caregivers can better maintain their own health and sanity. Changes don't need to be big to be effective.

Arts-based work—engaging with a creative process—works at a subconscious level to produce increased mental awareness and clarity. That's only one of the positive effects. The very act of creating helps change our brainwaves, slowing us down and causing a shift that brings us out of our day-to-day reality where we are concerned with *doing*, rather than just *being*. This is true even for passive activities such as listening to music or strolling through an art gallery. Movement through dance can have similar effects. Although there is a burgeoning area of research on the effects of art and creativity, it's not applied widely in academia. What a shame that is.

In this particular research study, called Arts in Home Care, each participant was required to create something—a piece of art, a photograph, a poem, mixed media images. It didn't matter what it was, as long as it represented some aspect of the caregiving experience. The respondent's choice of medium was up to them, as was the particular aspect of caregiving they chose to highlight. One person drew a picture depicting how both heart and hands are needed when giving care. Another did a collage of words she called "Word Rain," representing the feelings that fell from her eyes like tears. One wrote a poem about how tough it was growing up caring for her Mom who'd had a stroke when she was a teen. Each creation was used during the interview as a touchstone to further explore the caregiving experience. Where words are difficult, a work of art often prompts reflection and storytelling.

Donelle

It was a bright, snow-covered day in December when I arrived at Donelle's. As I walked down the long hallway toward her condo, I could already smell freshly brewed coffee. Donelle's home was open concept, neat, and tastefully decorated. A quilted wall hanging immediately caught my eye. She herself was immaculate, simply dressed in a blouse and slacks. Inviting me to sit on the sofa—she took the chair across from me—Donelle offered coconut cookies, along with tea or coffee. I chose coffee, even though it was early afternoon. The rich aroma was too inviting to pass up.

Donelle was the first respondent in this Arts in Home Care study and I was keen to hear her experience. We weren't long into our conversation when she took that stunning quilt off the wall and handed it to me for a closer look. The artistry was incredible. It turned out that she had made it in a workshop in Saskatchewan the previous spring. She hadn't planned on creating what she did. In fact, she told me how ugly it was when it started out. It just happened for her organically, over time.

She handed the quilt to me as she explained how she started by dying the fabric, describing in great detail how cathartic the whole process was. A world away from her day-to-day responsibilities, and from the worry about her husband, she could immerse herself in the project and forget about her reality. It didn't matter that she didn't know how she was going to proceed—things just started coming together.

"So, is this the piece that you created that day?" I asked.

"Yup," Donelle replied. "This is it."

I looked at her puzzled, "This is the one that you said was ugly?"

Donelle smiled, "Yup, this is it."

"Wow! Now, I would say this is beautiful. But I'll let you tell me about it because I'm interested in what it symbolizes to you."

Donelle said, "It looks better now than it did when I started, because there's a lot of over-coloring and over-dying on it to bring out the color. It doesn't have a lot of fancy embellishment. I mean, there were truly beautiful things that other people made that day; bright colors, glimmer, gold, happy-looking things, right? Whereas I wouldn't call this a happy piece. But it's how I was feeling." She paused and looked at the quilt in my hands.

"I created a yin-yang piece and that was a fluke, because I didn't do that on purpose. It came to be through just doing mandalas, playing with circles. For me, any kind of circle I did ended up being a two-sided image and that gave me an image to work from. As I continued, I realized that it truly expressed what was happening. That this yin-yang, that used to be a whole, is coming apart. And the one half of it, the red half," she pointed to the brighter, more patterned side, "is still organized, it reaches out and it's still together. The other half should have been that way. It should have been the complementary thing, but it's splitting apart."

I looked at the quilt as she talked.

Donelle continued. "And so, I mean, one half is me and one half is my husband. One half is me and how I'm staying in control to get through this situation, and the other half is me internally falling apart because I like to keep it together on the outside. But inside it falls apart—my brain is falling apart." She chuckled at herself, then she told me she just went with it, realizing that was how she was feeling at the time. "Ugly" was the word she kept using, but she continued with the colors regardless. It felt right.

This all made sense to me. Donelle's creative work sparked a knowing that was at a subliminal level until *something* helped it surface. She didn't even know her mind was in such a dark place until she started exploring her emotions through her quilting. She felt uncomfortable during that workshop, but it was only through the process of creating that she was able to experience the truth of her state of mind.

Committed to the workshop process, Donelle continued to study the fabric she'd created. She looked around at everyone else's eighteen-inch blocks and could see only bright colors. She felt that the only thing in common was that they were all eighteen-inch squares. As she saw the image coming forth from her blotchy cloth, she started to stitch into it. It became a circle, first shaping up on one side and gradually taking the same shape on the other side. However, each half of the circle was quite different—haphazard short stitches with no pattern, no story on the one side, with spaces, blanks, and stitches that were mottled brownish ochre and purple. The contrast on the other side of the cloth was striking. It was brighter, with light coming through the yellow, red, and orange hues in the center, like a shining sun. That's what I saw. On that side, her stitches were more even, curving in a flowing motion out from the focal point on that half of the cloth—the sun. Around and around, the stitches moved the eye, swirling outward like the sun's rays. A loosely curved "S" shape moved through the center. And there it was. Yin-Yang. Just like she described her life to me.

In future arts-based research studies and workshops, I would witness many caregivers uncover their subconscious knowing and become more deeply aware of their true emotions. In Donelle's case, this happened by creating the fabric she would use in her quilt. Following this study with Donelle and other family caregivers, I expanded my work to include workshops for therapeutic rather than research purposes. Donelle and other caregivers described the benefits they received from participating in the research in this way: that once they had the opportunity to reflect on the effects of caregiving, they could find strategies to cope with caregiving. Through my research, I was able to create workshops that would provide caregivers with similar experiences and benefits.

CHAPTER TWO

Resilience

"I will admit that there was a point the last New Year's Day, I woke up and I thought to myself, 'Oh here we go, year three of an indefinite sentence.'"
—Carol

Adapting to Change

'VE READ THOUSANDS OF PAGES of peer-reviewed articles, books, newspaper articles, and government documents on or about caregiving. The word "resilience" comes up in all of them, yet rarely is it explained or examined. "Resilience in caregiving" is one of those phrases that gets bandied about as if caregivers either have it or they don't, and they swim or sink accordingly. Nothing could be further from the truth.

Resilience is the ability to bounce back after being knocked down due to a setback or misfortune. It's a quality that helps us adapt to change and challenge in healthy ways, sometimes making us stronger than we were before. It's such a valuable tool that the US Army tested a resilience education program on more than a million of its people with an investment of $145 million with tremendous success in supporting its soldiers and commanders to deal better with trauma and combat.

I've interviewed and observed hundreds of caregivers over the years. They've told me what they did to manage their long days, how they viewed their situations, and the myriad ways they made themselves feel better while under prolonged stress. Each person I spoke with demonstrated tremendous resilience, but not once did they use the word or even recognize resilient behavior when I called their attention to it. So I took a closer look at the language they used when talking about their situations:

"I saw it as a positive experience."

"I had hope."

"I knew it wouldn't always be like this."

"It wasn't easy, but I'm stronger now."

Turns out that these caregivers were talking about resilience, whether they knew it or not.

Resilient people demonstrate characteristics such as a positive attitude, hope for the future, and a belief that they can bear obstacles, if not overcome them. Resilience allows us to flourish in the face of adversity—or at the very least, to endure. Resilient caregivers see their outlook as hopeful in spite of adversity. Resilience helps them continue day after day and manifests itself in a myriad of ways. Not surprising, as it is one of the most important concepts in family caregiving. It can mean the difference between coping or not, between acknowledging the small victories or feeling like a failure. Some caregivers may have more resilience than others; nevertheless, it is a skill—or set of skills—that can be learned.

Resilience Building

Resilience is how caregivers counter adversity and stress, but it can be hard to muster due to fear, anger, frustration, and hopelessness—all of which can become crippling. The ability to bounce back from adversity hinges on uncovering and untangling those underlying thoughts and shifting how we respond to them. We all have the ability to manage our thinking; in fact, it's about the only thing over which we do have control. What happens to us can be largely out of our hands. How we choose to react to a situation—that's entirely up to us.

Having studied human behavior for many years, particularly as it comes to dealing with illness, tragedy, stress, and family caregiving, I have observed that we can indeed train our brains. We *are* our thoughts. We cannot control what happens to us, only our response. We don't know what will happen tomorrow, or even in the next moment, and that's likely a good thing. But we can draw on the power of our thoughts for strength.

Fear can be paralyzing. Anger is uncomfortable, if not painful. Experiencing loss and feeling tremendous sadness amplifies the value in what is left behind. I'm not suggesting that we minimize our feelings. Resilience is not about denying our emotions; it's about having the ability to acknowledge them, sit with them, and move on. The great thing is that we can build skills to help us find our way out of a spiral of stress and create the opportunity to be more content, stronger, even happier. That's resilience.

Resilience Building

Skills	Attitudes	Behaviors
Practice conditions of enoughness	Positive self-talk	List what you do well
Know your capacity	Gratitude	List what you need to learn
Avoid negative thinking traps	Compassion for self	Be assertive, not passive nor aggressive
Look at best-case–worst-case and your likely scenario	Optimistic outlook	Respond actively and constructively to others
Acknowledge your feelings	Revel in your best, whatever your best is and know that's enough	Take action
Recognize your choices	Forgiveness	Ask for help
	Take charge attitude, maintain your power	Openly communicate
		Learn how to use humor

Carol and Todd

Carol and her husband, Todd, were caregivers for Todd's father, Max, who had multiple chronic diseases: congestive heart failure, COPD (chronic obstructive pulmonary disease), and atrial fibrillation. As his condition deteriorated, he became more frail and less steady on his feet, until he eventually fell in his home and broke his hip. It was then that Carol and Todd realized Max was no longer capable of managing safely on his own.

Max was adamant that he wasn't going to go to a nursing home. Carol and Todd didn't want that for him either, so together the couple decided the best option was for them to sell their house and renovate Max's home so they could live together. "We extended the house and created a large master bedroom with an ensuite, walk-in shower, and high-rise toilet to make things a little bit more comfortable for him. It also gave us all a bit of privacy," recalled Carol.

As a freelance writer, Carol was able to work part-time. Todd had a full-time job, so as Max's health deteriorated and his disease progressed, Carol was able to step in. "I handled his medications—made sure that he got those four times a day—did the cooking, the cleaning, meals, drove him to doctor's appointments and so on and so forth."

"Did you have any home care?"

"The home care we received was in the nature of respite care. When we first qualified, we received, was it…two hours or three hours, and that was about six months in?" She looked at Todd.

Todd confirmed, "Three hours every Wednesday."

"After about eight or nine months, he was being assessed by his home care nurses, and they said, 'Is three hours enough?' And it wasn't, so we got bumped up to four hours per week."

Max's health issues were primarily due to physical deterioration. He did have some mental deterioration toward the end, but he covered it up well.

On their one respite day each week, a care provider came from home care to give Max lunch that Carol had prepared. She would also assist him with showering and generally keep an eye on him while they "ran around and got a breath of fresh air, did the grocery shopping and so on," Carol said. "We only received one day a week. Because we were here full-time, that was all we were allowed. We would have wanted more and tried to get more, but that did not go well."

I hear that a lot. Families get just enough to get by, and getting by is not good enough. Home care programs strive to only give families what they need. Anything extra is perceived as a want and home care does not address wants. In fact, now the common mantra among home care administrators is to address *unmet needs*. I fully understand this from a health systems and efficiency perspective. When most of the services provided come under publicly funded health care, it's important to balance individual with societal needs. However, home care is woefully underfunded—whether in Canada's publicly funded provincial home care programs, in the United States through Medicaid or Medicare, and in the United Kingdom through the National Health Service; there just aren't enough resources to go around. The mantra often touted by policy-makers that "we will expand community care and provide more options for families outside of hospital care" is at odds with the reality that leaves family caregivers feeling defeated. When there is not enough outside support—health care dollars do not follow the client—the family must fill in the gaps at home.

Although there are private home care providers throughout the world, these can be expensive. They usually offer an hourly rate for various home care providers—nurses, health care aides, and others— in addition to offering public services through various government programs. They also typically provide home care through various insurance programs—both public insurance and private insurance, such as extended health care benefit programs. Of course, these options are available only to people with the coverage and there are eligibility criteria to meet; not everyone who has the coverage necessarily qualifies, so it is important to read the fine print. Health care is costly and home care is no different. On a private fee-for-service basis the cost can be prohibitive for many and in most instances, it is not sustainable over a long period of time.

From Analysis to Action

Family caregiving, like many of life's major stressors, can cause an existential crisis. While some caregivers may turn their most difficult experiences into catalysts for improved performance, others struggle. That's why it's important to take stock of our responses to external stimuli. That means encouraging a self-awareness about those cues and triggers that cause anxiety and stress.

Understanding our personal life view—the way we think about the world around us—can help us to better acknowledge our strengths and accept our weaknesses, and to help us move from paralysis to analysis to a plan of action (or reaction).

Carol and Todd were task-oriented and did what they needed to do to get through. They had mental fortitude and resilience. And they had each other, too. They benefited from their relationship, and we know strong and positive relationships play a significant role in resilience.

"Dad was still quite active," said Todd. "He continued going to meetings right up to a month and a half before he died. He stood up in front of thirty or forty people and spoke quite eloquently. So, in some cases, we had the best of situations…but there were the underlying tensions and the underlying problems which in retrospect, you think, 'Okay if we had done this, this and this, it would have made life a little easier. A lot easier.' But you learn that after the fact." Todd recognized some of the good things about their situation. Another aspect of resilience is the ability to be grateful and acknowledge what is working in your life.

Lessons from other caregivers can be helpful, too. Todd reflected that a week or two of out-of-home respite for Max would have given them the chance to take a holiday or relax at home. He knew they could have asked for more home care hours from a health care aide, but Max preferred Carol. He knows they could have worked harder to convince Max to accept outside help. They didn't realize how long their caregiving journey would last.

While it is often a good thing that we can't see through to tomorrow, let alone the next week or year(s), caregivers sometimes move forward naïvely thinking things will change, get better, or end soon and that affects decision-making—not always positively. Family caregivers want to do good by their loved one, so they put their own needs aside, which eventually affects their own health and well-being. When caregiving goes on for a long time, it needs a different approach than just coping and hoping. While it may be relatively easy for some caregivers to do certain tasks—physical care, home maintenance, and daily chores—on a short-term basis, over the long term it can lead to burnout, exhaustion, and even serious illness in caregivers themselves if there are not appropriate or sufficient supports in place. Some of these supports are external or targeted to the care recipient, such as more home care, but some also need to be specific to the caregiver—and not only take the form of respite but also coaching in resilience skills and coping strategies to build a caregiver's fortitude.

"Hindsight is 20/20," Carol agreed. After a moment she added, "There was an upside to this, by the way. I got involved in the community league movement and am now vice-president of the Edmonton Federation of Community Leagues." Carol said it was through bringing Max to his various groups that she met others in the community which prompted her to become more involved, something she wouldn't have done had she been engaged in her full-time work.

Many caregivers acknowledge how the new normal brought about by a caregiving role effects change in their lives. Carol's reflection illustrates the role of gratitude and appreciation, which also promotes resilience. The ability to recognize the paradox in the range of emotions active through caregiving helps build resilience: loss and gain, grief and gratitude, vulnerability and strength, change and stability. Resilience is about coping not only in the moment or following a stressful event or caregiving crisis; it is a personal quality that also helps caregivers bounce back from their whole caregiving experience.

Todd laughed. "All is not black."

"Our community league was right across the street and I got involved in self-defense."

Todd added, "You tend to look at the worst possible situation; you hear of something that's going well and you just ignore it. In all honesty, I think our situation was probably in the top one percentile of home care situations. I think we had the best possible world at the time." This positive outlook is a part of resilience. Our ability to see how our situation could be much worse helps us be thankful that it's not. We can always find people who have it better or worse than ourselves and recognizing that there are others in a caregiving role helps us feel less alone. In the midst of caregiving, thinking about the best case, worse case, and your true case can center you in reality and support resilience. Recognizing that you are not living your worst-case scenario can bolster gratitude. The way Carol and Todd used humor and looked on the bright side shone a light into their perspective—both are skills of resilient caregiving.

Todd and Carol believed they had it good; whether or not they did is not the point. It was their mindset that is important here. They acknowledged that the support they had, although not perfect, was valuable in helping them cope. They fully reflected on their situation and saw the positive. They were glad to have cared for Max in the way that they did.

Carol also felt that it was important to recognize Max's dignity, to see him for the man he was rather than a frail, older person who didn't have much to offer. She added, "That's the other thing. There's a tendency to infantilize the elderly as they become more infirm and it's not necessarily mental infirmity but even the physical infirmities, I think. I tried not to do that with Max." Recognizing the "other" is not something most caregivers have trouble with as they are so consumed with caregiving; however, remembering the positive things about the one you are caring for supports a positive attitude. Although it might not always be easy to recognize amid the stress of everyday caregiving, it is something that can be practiced.

"We made it work for three years. But I will admit that there was a point the last New Year's Day, I woke up and I thought to myself, 'Oh here we go, year three of an indefinite sentence.'" Carol acknowledged how harsh that sounded and admitted that the poignancy of the sentiment struck her the moment she thought it. She explained that it didn't mean she didn't want to be supporting Max, but that she did feel trapped. Acknowledging this helped her identify that she might need to do things to get her out of that mindset.

Todd was very quick to add, "No, but it's factual, and if we sugar-coat it, it doesn't do any good, either. That is reality. There's too much of the sugar-coating around caregiving, I find. People have to stand up and say, 'Look, I can't do this anymore.' Then, all of a sudden, alarm bells go off. If you just say, 'Well you know, I'm kinda tired, and yeah sometimes it's annoying...'" He shrugged. "But, 'Dammit, I can't do this anymore': that gets attention." He couldn't be more right. Recognizing limits promotes action, such as asking for help. Realizing that you have reached your capacity in some area does not mean you are a failure at caregiving. It means you have reached your limit with a certain aspect of caregiving. Reflecting on best-case–worst-case scenarios may help to view your own case more accurately. Once you see your situation more realistically, it can be a little easier to take all unhelpful thoughts of fear, failure, and over-whelm out of the equation, recognize your actual limit, see where you need support, and take action. Seeing your own reality more clearly guides you in knowing what you need to ask for. Resilient caregivers take action to improve their situation.

Todd and Carol's thoughtful reflection and their ability to look at their situation from a realistic perspective—and as Todd said, without sugar-coating it—reflected their resilience by grounding them in their actual reality. Being resilient isn't about being naïve or overly optimistic. It is about being able to do something about your situation. It is part of the catalyst for taking action to make things better—or at least make them better in your mind. It helps you to reframe your thoughts to reflect reality, rather than the worst-case scenario, which you probably are not actually living. At least not in every moment.

Bouncing Back

I saw various manifestations of resilience in all of the family care-givers who shared their stories with me, but mostly it wasn't obvious to them. Most caregivers understood the situation they were in and shared their stories because they wanted to make things better for others.

Resilient caregivers do seem to bounce back from difficult situa-tions better than others. But there is more to it than that. Resilience is a state of being that has a lot to do with being an effective caregiver and maintaining personal health and well-being. Yet, what struck me is that caregivers who are resilient don't recognize it, at least not until long after the fact when someone points it out to them.

In cases where resilient skills, attitudes, and behaviors were obviously present to me, the caregiver never named this as resilience, or at least not until it was pointed out to them. In situations where resilience was absent, I noted that skills in resilience would go a long way in supporting caregivers—not only as a way to help them cope better, but to encourage them to take action by requesting support for themselves or their loved one.

Resilience through Humor

Humor, positive psychology, and positive self-talk promote resiliency. My mother demonstrated those skills and behaviors. Recognizing the good qualities in Dad alongside her own limits helped her to deal with the paradox of living with strength and vulnerability—knowing when to laugh and when to cry, knowing when to just get on with it and when to seek help.

Watching Mom, I'd often wonder how she did it all. She did what she had to do for herself—carving out those little bits of time, saying what she needed and wanted—and for Dad. She was resilient, but that doesn't mean it was easy at all. She suffered health effects. She was exhausted and her blood pressure went up; both of these issues resolved within a few years after Dad died. Being resilient isn't Pollyanna-ish or without costs, but it is using your strengths to overcome what you are faced with without letting it overcome us.

Many caregivers find a way to draw on their strengths from within—they pull up their bootstraps and get on with it. Neither passive nor aggressive, they are assertive: grounded in their reality. Mom needed to feed Dad. She needed to take over his wound care and bowel routine. So, she adjusted each time something new arose. She didn't let a challenge or setback derail her for long. For her to not be assertive and take action, to not feed Dad, would mean he might choke and possibly end up in hospital with pneumonia, or have poorer nutrition or dehydration, or become malnourished or dehydrated, risking which leads to urinary tract infections, skin breakdown, and poor healing. Resilience allows caregivers to acknowledge their reality as it is and take action. In this way, resilience is not about our response to one particular challenge or moment in time, or doing everything perfectly all the time; rather, it is a way of being—a mindset, as well as a set of behaviors, that helps caregivers flourish rather than flounder and crash.

Carol and Todd used the little support they got to their advantage while doing the best they could building on their strengths. This was clear in my interview with them. They smiled a lot, and they chuckled from time to time when sharing their story. Max had died a few years before, and while it had clearly been a difficult time for them, they never lost their ability to look at things somewhat light-heartedly. A mark of resilience if ever there was one.

Todd laughed as he recalled a visit to the gerontologist. "There were some humorous stories. We were all quite happy Dad finally got in to see him and we had joked a little throughout the assessment. When the doctor finished his assessment with Dad, he looked at my father and he smiled and said, 'You know you've got the world by the ass.' Which was just the language that my father would under-stand and deal with. He said, 'You've got people looking after you, your meals are delivered to you. You've got everything.' Of course, Dad's looking at him and he says, 'You're right. I haven't got a care in the world!' So, there were little humorous incidents like that along the way and I believe they did help keep us moving in the right direction."

Penny, another caregiver, also told me humor helped her keep going through difficult times. She and her husband worked to keep their humor alive through jokes and using tongue-in-cheek phrasing. She said, "You know this one time, he came out of the hospital—I forget what he was going on about—he was being kind of cranky and fussy. Finally, I had had it, so I smirked at him and said, 'Shut up for a while, will you?' And he looked up at me and made a funny face and we both just started laughing. We would do that kind of thing. It's important to simply keep the humanness in it."

She went on to talk about how their little dog, Echo, also helps them. "She is such a hoot. She is fun to watch when we play with her. She keeps us laughing when we get her to do her tricks." Many people derive profound enjoyment from their pets, and caregivers are no different. Animals give them something else to focus on and provide immeasurable comfort.

A great deal of research has focused on the role of humor in resilience. We know the benefits of laughter for our health. Humor therapists in hospitals know that laughter does often come close to being the best medicine. This is one area where we don't need to rely on outside sources. Think about how you feel after a good laugh or even a chuckle. Even putting a smile on your face changes your mood and your voice. Try it: smile now. Feel your face change, feel that tug in your gut. It physiologically changes our state.

When I worked in home care, we were encouraged to answer the phone standing up and with a smile. The person we were talking to couldn't see what we were doing, but I bet they experienced it. Our voices were happier and stronger when standing up. And smiling added a note of warmth that callers were grateful to hear. People calling home care are often facing significant stress. Responding with a cheerful voice helps to engage the caller and promote calmness throughout the conversation. More than that, though, it's important to understand that we become our language and our thoughts. That smile can unlock positive feelings buried by difficult situations. Whereas negative views can foster more negativity, and so the cycle continues.

Humor can help break the vicious circle of destructive thoughts. It's a coping strategy and an effective technique in self-care. It can also be a deflector or an avoidance tactic, which may not be a bad thing either. The caregivers I know faced their situations head-on, but after doing that for twenty-four hours a day, seven days a week—well, sometimes you just need to look away.

I've heard caregivers joke about all sorts of things—like the time one of them put their cat in the basement away from a visiting nurse with allergies and forgot about it until that night, when they couldn't figure out where all the meowing was coming from. Another even laughed about how she kept putting her husband's urinal so far away from him he couldn't reach it to use it. She laughed at herself: "You keep doing the same old thing, the same old way, you get the same old result. I think he wet himself three times because of where I put it! Neither of us would notice in time and he would wet himself yet again. It was my fault," she said, "and it was a big chore to clean him up. You'd think I would have learned sooner! What do you do?" She shook her head at herself.

Another caregiver noted that it's often the little things that make you laugh. "As bad as dementia is, I just have to laugh every time I make Mom and myself sandwiches for lunch. Every time she says, 'We need a whole lot more. This will never feed all of those people!' I think she remembers all the times she made sandwich trays for our church functions. So, I just have to keep telling her. Most of the time she believes me but sometimes she thinks I am being mean and just don't want to feed those 'other people.' It's hard, but I have to laugh about it. What else can I do?"

Laughter can help us find a new way of living with adversity. Caregivers won't necessarily say, "Oh, that laugh I had the other day really helped me cope and build up my resilience." But they do say things such as, "It's better to laugh than cry all the time" or "You just had to chuckle, what else are you going to do?" I still hear my mother's voice saying "What do you want me to do? I could laugh or I could cry, and laughing is better. If I start crying, I might never stop."

I learned so much about the role of humor in resilience through listening to caregivers. I admire them for it and I think it is one of the things in caregivers' lives that keep them strong throughout their loved one's illness or infirmity. Most family caregivers and clients would rather be anywhere else than where they are. No one wants a chronic debilitating illness. No one wants a family member or friend to have one, either. However, when we find ourselves in such a situation, we deal with it— and humor can help get us through even the most difficult times.

Humor is not only about those moments in our personal lives that strike as amusing. We can find comic relief through external sources, too. Things like reading a story that gives us a good laugh, looking at the comic strips in the newspaper, or watching a comedy on TV are all ways we can bring humor into our lives. Although caregiving itself is often far from funny, when a humorous situation presents itself, laughing or chuckling and letting ourselves see the fun in it can help us maintain a healthy range of emotions. Laughter helps to strengthen resilience.

Resilience in Action

If I had to sum up what I observed about my mother's caregiving, it would likely be "resilience in action." Her behaviors are part of what makes a caregiver resilient—knowing and setting her own boundaries, being aware of her sense of self, not being a martyr. Mom would remind Dad that she was up with him at night, tell him when he was fine to wait on her for a time, that everything wasn't always such an emergency that she had to stop what she was doing and run to him. A non-resilient caregiver might not view reality the same way. They might be one to jump to conclusions, such as telling themselves they are a failure, that they should do more, that they need to sleep in the same room as the one they care for, even if only in a chair.

Mom told Dad that she had things she needed to do besides care for him, whether it was time in the morning for herself to shower, have a coffee and read the paper, or run errands. She was action-oriented and recognized that in order to get everything done she needed to get up at six. She knew herself well enough to know she needed some time for herself and for her it was those few moments of quiet in the morning before tackling the day.

I believe talking about what was going on with me and my siblings helped Mom to see the reality of her situation. Mom's relationship with us allowed her to be honest about her feelings—something important for all caregivers is to have a safe place to be open about *their* feelings and *their* needs.

This was Mom's routine as a full-time caregiver for Dad, 365 days a year over several years; it was easy to understand the personal resources and resilience she needed to deal with her caregiving role, day in and day out. She had to plan her day, focus on what needed to be done, and let other things go; she had to rest whenever she had the chance, learn to cope with people who disappointed her, and accept that most others would never be able to give Dad the kind of care she could. There was no time for much else in her life other than caregiving and planning around Dad's needs and his care aides' shifts.

I never would have called my mother's caregiving resilient until I was well into my program of researching and studying caregiving. Witnessing what it took others in her situation to provide constant care, day in and day out across several caregivers, brought the notion of resilient caregiving to light for me. Now I see it often. Being a resilient caregiver doesn't mean donning rose-colored glasses and maintaining a purely optimistic outlook. Resilient caregivers are realistic more than optimistic. They take each day as it comes and focus on what needs to be done. They maintain hope for the next day and know that they want to be there to do what they are doing rather than have someone else do it.

The drive to want to be the best caregiver to a parent or spouse might have been borne out of some obligation or the view that "my parent or my spouse looked after me," as well as the notion of "for better for worse" in spousal caregiving—but often caregivers just can't fathom leaving the job to anyone else. Of course, more than anything they wished their life was not like it is and that their loved one was healthy, but most believed this was the hand they were dealt and they would face it head-on. They do what needs to be done for their loved one, and advocate for what they need every day. They fight the good fight.

Although many caregivers say they couldn't keep going day after day without support from others, either care providers or family and friends, their stories demonstrate resilience. In spite of the fact that sometimes people let them down, it can be difficult getting information and answers, and there are shortcomings within systems intended to help them, somehow they find a way to keep on giving care.

Building Resilience: Journal Practice

Time commitment: Five to ten minutes

Take out a pen and paper and consider what you are struggling with.

Write down one thing that comes to mind.
Ask yourself what you can do about it. Keep it simple. Try to avoid those things you cannot control. If they come into your mind write them on another scrap paper and put it someplace else, write it in a different part of your journal, or write it and put a box around it. This is about identifying what YOU can control.

Write down your answers. Don't judge yourself. Don't overthink. You might have other concerns to list; repeat the process for each one.

Do this every day. Even if you're documenting the same feeling.

This is a practice. That's why you do it every day. Practice builds resilience.

You become your thoughts.

You may take action on your thoughts today or tomorrow. You may not. But this practice is about writing down solutions and reminding yourself about what you can do to take charge of your thoughts, beliefs, and feelings around a particular problem.

Practice every day. Be committed to coping well.

CHAPTER THREE

Change, Loss, and Grief

"I'm like a widow with a husband. But it's even worse because he's here."
—Olivia

WHEN I FIRST STARTED RESEARCHING family caregiving, I thought I had a good sense of the issues. Not only had I witnessed my mother take care of my father for twenty-two years, but I had worked directly with clients and family members as a home care nurse and administrator for over twenty-five years. As soon as people heard what field I was in, they were quick to tell me about their situation. I listened to countless stories on the street, in line at the grocery store, and over dinner. People told me about looking after a mother who had since died, a father who had a chronic disease, a grandmother looking for long-term care. I heard so many scenarios from adult children of all ages and I quickly learned that grief and resilience reside together.

This work, and these stories, were things I thought I knew something about. However, when I began to interview people in depth, it didn't take long to realize that each case was much bigger and far deeper than I had initially thought. As a researcher, I was struck by the vastness of the issues intimate family caregivers faced and the wholly consuming nature of the role. Early on in my research studies I asked myself how I could have missed the essence of the caregiving relationship and the significance of what these people were going through. They were riding a very large wave of change, loss, and grief. And in most cases, things did not get better.

That was certainly true of my own family. My father's illness devastated us all. He lost the physical ability to do things he wanted to do and, over time, the essence of who he had been. Mom lost her husband and best friend. We lost our father, bit by bit. It was relentless, always losing ground. There would be good days, for sure, or times when progression slowed, but overall it was a downward trend.

"That's not the man I married," my mother said to me one day, shaking her head. "My God. Imagine your father getting this disease. He was always so healthy and so strong. Look at him. He is so small. We had twenty good years of marriage and then it's gone. Who would have thought this is where we'd be? It's like I'm married to an old man."

Although Dad was never confused in the way people with various dementias are, he became mentally dull and had difficulty processing information. At first the changes were slow. He went from walking to occasional stumbling, to falling, to falling more. From there he moved to a half cane, then to a full cane, then to needing assistance to stand. Then he required a wheelchair. After that he was confined to bed. Meanwhile, we saw a decline in his mental status. The once vital man who loved to engage in conversation lost the ability to find the right word. He became dull, as if his thoughts were jumbled. He relied on clichés for a time, smiling and nodding as if to follow a conversation. Toward the end, he would mostly doze off. With each gradual change came an unavoidable withdrawal from his own life, and ours. We knew it was only a matter of time, and so in many ways we were waiting.

Loss and grief are real phenomena in caregiving that sometimes don't get their due attention. Caregivers learn to live with ambiguity both in terms of the functional ability and health status of the loved one for whom they are caring. The trajectory of the way they experience loss is not usually known, particularly in the case of dementias when the dependent individual is physically present but not there mentally—the person they knew is gone. Physical decline can have a similar effect, even while mental capacity remains. Loss of function, loss of social life, and increased isolation result in sadness and grief over all that was expected from life but is no longer possible.

Caregivers experience grief in several ways and sometimes over many years. They grieve over ambiguous losses, but also over the impending death of their loved one, regardless of how far away that may be. Anticipatory grief happens when the person we love is still here, but not quite or not in the same way. Anticipatory grief can be a long stage of mourning for some and also brings other emotions with it—guilt, anger, sadness, fear. While sadness is often about the loved one being cared for—how they are living, their pain, disease process, and hurt—the grief is the caregiver's burden. Often, they don't talk about it as it doesn't tend to be considered amid the day-to-day caregiving duties, but rather it comes up in quiet moments or in the middle of the night. Caregivers usually don't want to share their grief with their loved one because they don't want them to feel worse: Their day-to-day caregiving is usually focused on wanting to make their loved one feel safe, secure, and happy. Anticipatory grief may be experienced as an undercurrent—a knowing that it is always there or as an episodic event when the sadness becomes overwhelming and thoughts of death are more present, bringing up feelings of guilt and even anger for thinking that perhaps death might be better for one's loved one and oneself, and then feelings of anger that they are experiencing such loss and sadness, and at themselves for thinking such a thing.

Grief is not experienced in a linear manner, nor do we all experience the various stages of grief—the common ones being shock, denial, anger, sadness/depression, bargaining, and acceptance—in the same way. In family caregiving grief is often present, but it comes and goes with changes and everyday moments over time. We don't go through one stage only to be done with it; rather, we circle through the stages many times. The symptoms of grief can be physical, emotional, social, and spiritual, and felt to greater and lesser degrees.

I often grappled with feelings of anger and sadness during the years Dad had MS. I resented his decline and the loss of what I counted on him for most—advice. My Dad was a kind and rational man. I was used to getting guidance from him and he was always, always, there for me. I always believed he'd be there for me. I guess I took him for granted. He was, after all, my father.

When I was in my mid-twenties, I finished my graduate degree in nursing and moved to the Canadian prairies where I accepted a job as a Nurse-In-Charge, with responsibility for the health units in four First Nations communities. I loved my job—focusing on public health, learning about what made these communities unique, supporting and leading my staff, feeling that I might make at least a little difference—but I hated being so far away from home. I went home to visit about every six months, mainly because of my Dad's health, which was a little worse on each trip. More than feeling obligated, I *wanted* to see him as much as I could.

On one particular visit, I was feeling distressed about a human resources problem with a few employees. I was new to management in a rural area; my peers, whom I might normally have run things by, were in other communities. Dad and I were chatting about this and that is when it occurred to me that he might be able to share some insight, given his past experience as a manager.

"Dad, I have these two staff who are driving me crazy."

He looked at me as I continued.

"They don't seem to respect my gentle cues as to what is expected. I think I need to openly discuss the problems with them. I don't expect it will go well as they are still testing me. Carol, the nurse before me, did the job for twenty-some years. Based on what I hear, she was pretty lenient. Things could be run a lot better. But because Carol was there for so long and they got away with so much, it's not going to be easy."

"That's right," Dad said. "You will have to think about how you deal with them." He likely said something like "useless bastards," but I can't quite recall.

I went on. "They don't bother doing home visits if they don't feel like it. They show up for work an hour or more late. Sometimes they withhold information and I honestly don't know if it's because they can't be bothered, don't think it's important, or just want to trip me up. They talk endlessly with their friends or family who show up in the clinic, even taking them into their office and closing the door for a chinwag—sometimes for long stretches at a time—all while other patients are waiting to be seen. They don't care. I often have to knock and basically tell them to get back to the clinic because we have a line-up. Sometimes—and get this—they might not even bother coming back to work after lunch!"

"I get so damn frustrated. They really should be terminated so we can bring in some new people who *will* work!"

Dad looked at me with compassion and interest, nodding all the while.

"Other than that, I love the job. I think we're getting on top of lots of things. The Chief seems to trust me and he likes what I'm doing. In fact, I get great support from him and some of the counsellors. Maybe that rubs Arlene and Sue the wrong way. One of the biggest problems is that there are so many hoops to jump through and processes to follow within government that it will take me a least a year to enact any progressive disciplinary action. I don't think anything has been dealt with in recent years, even though the problems were there and I see notes on their files where Carol had initiated something. But she never followed through."

I felt myself getting worked up at the telling of the story, so I decided to stop talking and hear what my Dad had to say. His response is vivid in my mind.

"I'm sorry, dear," he said raising his head to look at me. "I don't know what to say to you. I can't think through something like that anymore."

It took me a moment to comprehend what he was saying. Time seemed to slow.

He shook his head from side to side again. "I'm just no good to you on that. I don't know what to say." He glanced out the window then turned back to me and smiled lamely. My heart broke a little more that afternoon.

MS is a horrible disease. It doesn't cause dementia *per se*, but it sure affected Dad's ability to process information.

"Don't worry, Dad. It's hard for you and I was telling you lots and not necessarily in order. Don't worry about it. It was good to share it with you, anyway."

We went on to talk about something else. I forget what we moved on to—it likely wasn't significant—but what I do remember is a feeling of shock and wanting to cry. He was failing more each time I went home. My strong, capable father was losing so much ability, even to participate in conversation. And this was still relatively early on in his disease.

I think about that afternoon and our conversation often, especially when I reflect on losses that other caregivers have experienced. It was a turning point for me when I realized the impact of his disease on our lives. Over time, I accepted it. I was mostly sad about it, and I regularly vacillated from anger to acceptance—mostly because we talked openly in our family. We acknowledged the sadness, but we also talked about what could have, and should have, been. I think the openness among my parents and siblings are what made all the difference for me—that, and the love in our family, though not the saccharine kind. We are blessed with so much love, but we have also had differences of opinion over the years.

My mother always told us how important it was to make amends with each other from a very young age—actually, she made us! We never got away with "not speaking" in our house. Someone was usually more in the wrong and to not talk and apologize made everything worse and uncomfortable. Talking about differences and apologizing for hurtful things said is not always easy but—to me—it is much worse to do otherwise. Now that I am older, I see that as one of the best gifts my parents gave us as a family. I have a fantastic relationship with each of my siblings and I feel blessed with each of them. The close relationship I have with my siblings is often pointed out to me first by friends, and also by colleagues once they come to know my story. I believe how we are with each other today is, in part, a result of my father's illness. Of course, there are many families affected by animosity or fractured relationships. When caring for someone who is ill and infirm, though, love and support can make all the difference. Sharing sadness and grief with others who understand invariably eases the burden.

Katarina

Katarina understood that loss and sadness are part of the caregiver's journey, particularly with aging parents, but that knowledge hasn't made the experience of looking after her mother any easier. She wrote a poem in an arts-based research project I was leading. Here is the last stanza of her poem, *Roles Reversed*.

Stubborn, she holds her credentials
As life-giver high, even as I dish out her food,
And listen, good girl again, as I guide her feet
Into her shoes and spell out her conversation
On the palm of her hand,
Tears burning behind my eyes
Which see for the two of us
On this sunset-flooded journey.

Each time I read this I am struck by the sense of loss Katarina must have been feeling through her sadness. I heard some version of what she expressed in her poem from many adult children looking after frail or aging parents. Although change, loss, and grief are felt by all of the caregivers I spoke to, no two people experience these things in the same way. I found that their experience largely depends on the nature of their relationship with their parent as well as their respective ages and stages of life.

Katarina began to support her mother over twenty years ago when she started to lose her sight due to a progressive degenerative disease. Her mother has now lost all of her vision and is also hearing impaired to the point where they use touch sign language to communicate and a special modulation device on her phone so she can hear speech. Katarina recited her poem to me as she did to her mother, using the phone, as that was the only way she could share it with her.

Katarina lives downstairs in her mother's house so she can be there for emergent and urgent needs. Although her mother is also supported by her husband—a man she met in a support group who also has the same condition but is much more independent. They do not have any outside support other than a home cleaner. Katarina provides five to twenty hours a week of care and support to her mother. She told me that getting the right kind of outside help can be challenging but with the home cleaner and the care she provides it is mostly working.

"Trying to get help and being worried about them at the same time is a little tough. At the same time, I am monitoring my own reactions because it's very easy to get frustrated when you're dealing with somebody who has a disability and is related to you. I find with strangers, if you are in a paid job or even volunteering, generally the boundaries are more set. So, that makes a difference.

"It really does affect the relationship in terms of how you are treated and how you treat the person. The caregiver needs to know their own emotional reactions to what's going on. I find the emotional aspect of the whole affair the hardest. There is so much emotion involved when it's your parent because you're watching them deteriorate so to speak and…" she paused. "It can be quite sad."

"Yes, it is," I agreed, "and it's not always easy to think about our own state through caregiving when some days can be busy or overwhelming. What helps you?"

"Well, my mother and I are both creative. We have always had a connection through that. I am a writer and a poet, she is an artist. In fact, she was a very talented artist."

"I see. Did that have anything to do with the colors you mention in your poem? I found them to be so vivid and specific." I read from her poem:

In the not-too-distant past she groomed me,
Taught me to read the shades of pencil crayons—
Burnt umber, sienna, turquoise, magenta—
Held my hand as we crossed the street…

Katarina nodded as she replied. "I liked the sounds of those colors. I think also that because my mother used to do artwork— she took many art lessons before she became disabled—even when

I communicate with her, I try to describe things in terms of artist's colors so that she will have a more vivid picture in her mind of exactly what shade the dress is that she's going to put on or something like that. It helps a lot."

"Oh, yes. I can understand that. You lived with those colors daily. When you're describing something to your Mom, it's not just pink, it's a particular shade of pink."

"Right, because she was so talented. Colors had to be specific in her art. I guess it was one of the ways I kept her former world alive for her, too. It was meaningful for both of us."

I understood her poem on a different plane now. I was touched and felt a pang of sadness and loss for her. We do pay attention and work hard to preserve our parent's former lives for them. Maybe that's part of why I would often ask my father so much about his work and how he dealt with his employees. It was something that tangibly connected us for just a little bit longer.

"You used a beautiful phrase, *sunset-flooded journey*. That really resonates. Can you describe that phrase in terms of what it means to you?"

"I was thinking about how, as you get older, those years are some-times referred to as the sunset years—that kind of thing. I was going for a colorful image with that thought to express that I'm not getting any younger, either, even as my Mom gets older, more frail, more dependent. We know where things are heading. We're both getting older and are on this journey together."

"I immediately pictured the beautiful sunsets at my family home over the harbor: orange, magenta, yellow. Sad, but peaceful."

She nodded. "Yes, you got it—that's it."

"You said earlier that you learn to appreciate everything—the people coming in, like the home cleaner, or the nurse who comes to give her a flu shot and things like that. You said you are pleased with her medical care and her physicians, but when you think about support from home care you mentioned something." I quickly looked down at my notes. "You said, *No matter what, I don't want her to lose her independence any more than she already has. I want to keep that.* Can you tell me more about that?"

"I think it's very important to her because she really thrives on her independence and it's very difficult for her to have to rely on other people. She recently started to suffer from depression because of losing her hearing on top of losing her sight. She started on anti-depressants, which I didn't like but she needed them. Losing more of her senses is very traumatic, and then having to rely on other people—even me and her husband—leads to frustrations."

"She recently started talking about her death: she wants to pass away at home type of thing, when she gets older. But she is also pretty frail. It's very important to her that she come and go as she pleases in order for her to be happy."

"I can understand that."

"She is constrained so much by her disability. There is a level of support she needs and it's growing. I try to give her what she needs but not be too overbearing. It's sad watching her like this. I think we are figuring it out. At least for now until something else changes."

"Yes, I hear that from a lot of people—the balancing required. Most caregivers of aging parents want the relief of people providing our parents with appropriate support, yet still helping them maintain their independence and help themselves as long as they can in whatever means they can, rather than having others do what they can otherwise do. So I relate to what you're saying. How old is your Mom?"

"She's sixty-six."

"That is not very old."

Katarina nodded. She looked pensive, "But she is very frail."

The anticipatory grief Katarina alludes to in her writing is part of the new state of normal brought about through caregiving. Although most accept it as they deal with the day to day, it does not negate the emotional toll of a looming and sad outcome. Accepting this reality is one of the things that needs to occur before we come to terms with it.

The Spousal Difference in Loss and Grief

People who take care of their spouses often talk about how challenging it is to cope with the loss of the one they love while they're in the midst of taking on a caregiving role. While many of the stories I heard were filled with practical wisdom and heartbreaking recollections, the one thing every spousal caregiver told me was that the person they were now caring for was no longer the person they married.

Jeanette

Jeanette was a participant in a collage-making workshop. The group, which I facilitated, encouraged caregivers to create art that reflected their experiences as intimate family caregivers. Each project was unique; many were exceptional. Some collages were filled with pictures of food, representing how much planning and consideration went into caring for their loved ones, as well as the significance of shared family meals. Others used pictures that expressed hobbies like gardening or painting, things that were important to their self-care. There were images of planes, trains, and faraway places signifying happy memories of trips taken. In some cases, these images stood for the sadness of unfulfilled dreams.

At the time of the workshop, Jeanette had been caring for her husband John, a former teacher, for a few years. John had Alzheimer's disease. Although she had been told his condition would not likely progress too quickly, it was, in fact, progressing rapidly. John and Jeanette were in their late sixties. While sharing her collage of images of a couple baking and another of people around a table (representing the support group she finds she now relies on), Jeanette made several comments about losing, or having lost, her husband. She sometimes compared him to a child. This mirrored the little old man metaphor my mother used in reference to my father. Jeanette shared her feelings of loss without prompting.

"I have to say, 'John, be sure you go to the bathroom,' because he has been known to go in the bush. It's like a little child, just constant. I have to tell him where the toothbrush is. He's physically capable of doing it but I have to say, get the toothbrush, put the toothpaste on, turn on the water. I had no idea there were that many steps to *every* single thing that he has to do. So, we brush our teeth, then after that it's okay, gotta shave." She described her current frustration about his reluctance to shower. "Like right now, I am giving him until Monday to have a shower. If he hasn't had his shower by Monday that's it, I'm phoning and they [home care] have to do something about this because it's been one week today. It's the longest he's ever gone. He brushed his teeth once this week, too, and that was to go to..." She paused. "Usually if we have an appointment, he'll do it. This is the second time he's gone to the doctor where he wouldn't shower. No shower, no shave, just brushed his teeth. This Tuesday was so bad that I thought I'd either have to go alone or take him in his house-coat, but as it turned out he got dressed and brushed his teeth."

"It's all difficult. It's hard, it's draining. It really is like having a child that you can't discipline and he gets angry and he gets violent and there's nothing I can do about it. We had a sign that acted as a cue for him. We still have that sign on the fridge that says, 'Only loving touch and no throwing,' but now it doesn't work because I guess he feels there's no consequence, so what the heck, you know? I guess the most difficult," she paused, "to be sure, is his hygiene. I have a hard time with that. I think about the future, what I've heard about how things could go, and I think, 'Oh my God, please, please don't let this happen to John, that he'll always know where the toilet is.' I'm contemplating getting one of those seat bidets. Maybe he won't know how to use it but," she paused, "because sometimes when I send him to the day program, he has wet ones, like portable wipes, in his back pocket but he has come home and with his shorts and I can tell, the smell, he didn't wipe. So I guess that might be the hardest thing is the hygiene. He was never like that."

John's loss of his ability to take care of his own personal hygiene was a concrete daily reminder of what Jeanette had lost and what they had lost as a couple—their relationship as they knew it. Over a short period, John went from being an independent partner to Jean's dependent. I heard the sadness in her voice as she shared the changes she was grappling with—new challenges almost every day.

Jeanette talked about her sadness and loneliness, as well as the lack of communication in their relationship. She recalled trying to talk with him about getting their fence repaired. "I guess that's why the fence has been delayed, it's because there's no feedback and I have a hard time with that, like he doesn't know. I say, 'Well should we get this guy, that guy?' He says, 'Oh, it's up to you,' or he just gets mad and says, 'I don't care.' It's like I am alone. I *am* alone. I have a body here with me, that's it. It's not the husband I married, absolutely."

Jeanette pointed to some other images she used in her collage. One was an image of people at a funeral. "Well, that's definitely John," she said. "It's an ongoing funeral."

I have heard many descriptors for the experiences of being a spousal caregiver and while most spouses express a sense of profound loss, Jeanette's funeral metaphor jolted me. But after a funeral there is a time of grieving when a spouse can typically reflect on the years gone by, the good times and the hardships, too. There is tremendous sadness, but there is resolution, an opportunity to take stock and consider how to move on. Widows and widowers need to relearn how to cope on their own and that can be hard, especially when the marriage has been a long one. But there's a difference in outlook when a partner has died, especially when the remaining spouse has carried the responsibility of being an intimate family caregiver. Suddenly, the goal is no longer making it through the day, but making a life.

Caregivers move through phases of grief throughout their caregiving role. It is a myth that we only grieve over death. Caregivers grieve and are bereaved over many of the losses experienced and for the person engaged in long-term caregiving, grief and loss are ongoing and often cyclical. The infamous grief expert Elizabeth Kubler-Ross first identified the five classic stages of grief in 1969—denial, bargaining, anger, depression, and acceptance. They were widely adopted for many situations dealing with loss. However, they are not linear, are not the only reactions to grief that a person will experience, and they aren't a one-shot deal. The grief process isn't a start-to-finish process and many stages are experienced more than once over time. In fact, many of us might be reminded often of what grief is like as feelings of anger, sadness, and even acceptance come back into our mind long after our loved one has died. There are other reactions as well such as fear, guilt, sadness, and shock and disbelief to name a few. There may be accompanying physical symptoms as well such as GI upset including nausea and diarrhea, insomnia, loss of appetite, high blood pressure, and immune deficiencies for example. Even the renowned expert said these five stages were never intended to be neat tidy boxes to contain our reactions to loss. Each of the reactions, or stages, she described are some of the reactions many people experience when faced with losses and particularly a death. However, losses are not all the same and nor are people the same and so our reactions to grief are as unique as ourselves. While life might sometimes feel like a funeral, the end is not in sight and may not be for a long time. That is what makes it exhausting and makes it feel like a never-ending journey.

Grief is difficult. It takes a lot of energy.

"It's just, you feel alone," Jeanette told me. "You have no partner...I've lost companionship. I've lost communication. I've lost shared activities and hobbies. We did so many things together. The intimacy, I really miss that. I ask for hugs, but it's not the same."

It's not the same. If ever there was a phrase to depict the trials of caregiving, that would be it.

"I'm overwhelmed. It's all this," she said, as she pointed to another section of her collage. There was a fair bit of white space and she said, "This presents us with a big zero. There's no life left anymore, there's none, it's gone. The stress level is high. I'm sad, I'm overwhelmed, I'm frustrated." She pointed to the different words she made out of letters torn from a magazine—On-going funeral, No support, Helpless, Fear, and Life is over—before pointing at one of the few images she used in her collage. "This is my one joy," she tapped the picture, "this little dog here represents my dog."

Therein lies the key to getting through: know what makes you happy and a little more at ease. That list of things is also as unique as the caregiver and as unique as their situation. What works for one won't work for all. Sometimes what a caregiver needs one day won't be the same the next. Sometimes, it's trial and error to find something to be happy about and sometimes it may be best to sit with your emotions for a while, or write about them, or remember better times or think about the future.

Working Through Grief

There are many experts (researchers, therapists, psychologists, counsellors) who specialize in grief and bereavement. Your local library will be able to offer a range of titles dealing with loss and grief, and websites of many caregiver organizations can often provide useful links and resources.

Additionally, these strategies can be employed on your own. This is not an exhaustive list but is intended as a starting point. If you are experiencing persistent depressive symptoms, sadness that won't let up, or thoughts of self-harm, seek immediate help from your physician or health professional. It is available.

Things to try:

Join a support group or your local caregiving society.

If you practice a particular faith, seek out your minister, priest, or pastor.

Talk to a therapist or counsellor.

Try writing down your feelings by journaling.

Make a list of all the things you enjoy:

What did you love to do at another time in your life, even as a child or a teen?

List any long-forgotten hobbies.

What brings you joy today?

List everything you can and then ask yourself what you would like to do again. You will likely have a vast array of activities, both active (like going for a walk) and more passive (like listening to music or watching a particular kind of television show).

Pursue learning something new, independently, online, or in a class.

Practice mindfulness and deep breathing. If you don't know where to start, try a yoga class (either online, which may be more convenient, or in person, to get out and practice in a community of people).

(*Continued*)

Talk to someone—other family members, including your children or siblings, or friends. There are caregiver groups and groups for bereaved caregivers online, as well.

Finding something you find helpful and that you enjoy will take intentional effort and trial and error. Go easy on yourself and remember that trying is the point. Give it time and praise yourself for trying.

Olivia

"It's completely different," Olivia said. "I'm like a widow with a husband. But it's even worse because he's here." She appeared to be lost in thought for a moment before continuing. "You know, we always used to do things together, we travelled together, we cooked together, we gardened together, we did everything together. Now I'm essentially by myself and the people we used to associate with, especially family, they've just…they no longer associate with us."

This wasn't that different from Jeanette's metaphor of a funeral.

Olivia's husband also had Alzheimer's disease. She provided his personal care as well as took care of all household chores, financial management, and necessary home repairs. Even though she had some help from paid caregivers through the home care program, she said the more she took on the role of caregiver, the more she lost her role as wife. When asked about support from her children she replied, "It's not the kind of support that I had from my husband…but they do support me very, very much. So, I've got my son and daughter-in-law and then yeah, my two caregivers."

I knew what she meant. My siblings and I were a support to Mom, but we couldn't replace Dad. Nobody could.

It is the significant change in the relationship between a husband and wife that makes spousal caregiving unique. When Jeanette was reflecting on this with me, she said, "Our lifestyle changed—everything about our life together." The support and reassurances she used to get from her husband—that things will be better tomorrow—are no longer there and she missed it. Their planned future will not be happening. She felt so much loss yet was helpless to do anything about it. "We used to get all dolled up. We don't dress up anymore. We used to love to dress to the nines and go somewhere. It's just all gone."

Oliva said something similar. Even though her children were there to help her when she needed help, or do things with her like go out for dinner or go shopping, it wasn't the same. Olivia missed her spouse—her partner in life.

Patricia

Patricia had a happy demeanor, in spite of what she was dealing with. It can be difficult for caregivers to maintain a positive stance while they are coping with loss and grief through caregiving; nevertheless, she displayed a positive attitude. At the collage workshop, Patricia showed her artwork, pointing to the words she copied from the Garth Brooks song, *The Dance*—"We had a great dance and I'm glad I took the chance."

"That's the way I feel. I wouldn't want to have missed it. It's not easy and I certainly don't like it. But he was my husband and always my rock. We had a good life. Things are different now—definitely a sadder time. Now it's my turn to be his rock."

Vic and Patricia were a solid, loving couple. In Patricia I saw such resilience, dedication, and a positive attitude—more so than I see in most who are dealing with the gradual decline and eventual loss of their spouse. Being so up close and personal with families when they are working their way through grief causes me to think about how I would handle things. I reflect on my own relationship with my husband. I pray that when the time comes, I will be as strong and loving as some of the caregivers I witness.

Patricia and Vic had three children, two boys and a daughter who is a nurse. She described them as a close family and strong in their faith; something that helped her cope with actual and anticipated losses while caring for Vic through his decline and their changed future. Several caregivers spoke of their faith and often mentioned praying specifically as something that helped them accept what they were dealing with. Many find that their faith eases their burden through the knowledge that, in spite of everything, they can still give some of their trouble to God or other deity of their choosing. Patricia and Vic had always been involved with their church in the various cities they lived in, and this continued after they retired and moved to a lakeside home in British Columbia. Vic's health started to decline with a barrage of serious health problems and hospitalizations.

Patricia described the year before his final diagnosis. "In a one-year time frame, we dealt with a lot. It seemed that we were faced with something new—but never good—to cope with every month as our life slowly dissipated over that year. It started with open heart surgery for a valve replacement. On his third day home, he developed a hernia at the surgical site and had to have emergency surgery. At the same time, he developed a very high heart rate—atrial fibrillation—so he was a very high-risk surgery. I thought I was going to lose him that time, but he survived. A few months later, he needed a cardioversion and that was unsuccessful. Two months later, he was doing much better but after a night of curling, shortly after he came home, he collapsed—unconscious. I called the ambulance and he was admitted with tachycardia—a rapid heartbeat. They diagnosed an abdominal aneurysm during one of his surgeries and because of his condition they took a 'wait and see' approach. I honestly didn't know what to hope for—more time with him watching him deteriorate with every episode, or a peaceful ending to all of it. Then I felt guilty! It was a tough year. *Every time* he went into the hospital, I thought I was losing him. You could say I had some dress rehearsals for his death that I could have done without—and so could he."

"Two months after the tachycardic episode he was beginning to feel good again. He was hiking in the park behind our house and slipped and fell. He didn't remember walking home but he said he was okay. I knew enough to watch him closely. Initially, he seemed to be fine and then he began a rather rapid decline—mentally. He often became agitated and one night I couldn't stand it any longer—this was new for Vic. I called the ambulance yet again. They found a huge blood clot on the left frontal lobe of the brain and had to operate. He came through it, but he deteriorated rapidly and was diagnosed with dementia. I was shocked—surely this wasn't right. But, I knew, deep down—it runs in his family. Out of ten children, five have it—three have died and he and his younger brother are both now living with it. So that's the medical history, that's where we are."

I felt drained for Patricia. I thought of many of the caregivers who went through similar complicated medical episodes before settling into a new normal—a life of caregiving and dealing with the loss of their loved one, a little at a time—knowing the only outcome would eventually be death. I knew it was a trying period for many of them. Shortly after that year ended, Patricia and Vic decided they needed to move to be closer to their adult children and grandchildren for more support for both of them. By the time Patricia came to my workshop, Vic was only a few years into his dementia diagnosis and they had been back in Alberta for a little under a year.

Patricia saw the advertisement for the workshop in the local paper and signed up right away. She said, "For the first time in the last two years, I felt alive. I felt alive at the seminar and then when we talked, I just felt all the things that are important to me now were there in my collage. Dr. Frank, our geriatrician, said caregivers need to know what makes them feel creative or what inspires them. The workshop was the first time I've felt that since Vic got sick, so it was an unexpected gift. Yeah, it really was a gift."

As she talked about her collage, Patricia said it was a gift because it helped her see that although they'd moved to a new normal there were still things she could feel grateful for. It helped her get back to her more positive self and appreciate the loving life they led. "What came to me through the process, and what I tried to portray is how lucky we've been in love. Love being a very generic term but," she laughed, "our relationship, well, over the years we built it and worked it well. This will be our fifty-third anniversary this September and I think that after that many years you realize that what you thought love was when we were young was really commitment. I don't think there's much difference between the two. We were lucky."

"I like to write and read. My favorite, and it hangs over our bed, is the poem that Elizabeth Barrett Browning wrote, '*How do I love thee? Let me count the ways.*' She had a great love affair with Robert Browning. I thought he was the most romantic of the two with, '*Grow old along with me, the best is yet to be. The last of life for which the first was made.*' And so '*Grow old along with me, the best is yet to be*' also hangs over our bed. I was going to use that as the theme for my collage, but I don't think the best is yet to be anymore. We lost so much, so quickly, and neither of us was ready for that. It's hard to see that and accept it. So I thought the words, '*I'd do it all again, rather take the chance than to have missed the dance,*' were much more appropriate for my collage. It really helped me to get the words down."

Recognizing her choice—that she would do it again—gave her strength. It was a similar refrain I heard from many caregivers, men and women alike, and regardless of the relationship between caregiver and the one for whom they were caring. Many said this with conviction. They easily recognized the tragedy of the situation, but they wouldn't have wanted anyone else to be in their place. As hard as it is, they are happy to have had the chance to care for their loved one. I never fully grasped how strong this conviction was until this past year, in the midst of editing this book, when I became my husband's caregiver through his diagnosis of aggressive prostate cancer, surgery, and follow-up care and appointments. The first thing I thought was, "I don't want to be here in this place—at all." But, during that time, I was also happy that it was me in the role of caregiver, able to do whatever I could to support him, care for him, and ease his pain and discomfort any way I could. I knew I did not want anyone else to do it—even home care.

Patricia explained, "I added all the pictures of the sports up there because that's who my guy was. Whether it was biking, whether it was golfing or skiing or hockey, or curling. All of those things were who he was as a person. I'm not an athlete but I'm a gall-darn good cheerleader," she laughed. "I was always there to cheer him on and I think that he would agree with that. I was trying to fit as many sports in there as I could. We used to bike quite a bit. I loved the time through our forties and fifties, when we did a fair amount of biking together."

"Just the other night when our granddaughter was visiting us, she said, 'I want to find a guy like my grandpa someday,' and I said, 'Yeah, we've had a pretty good dance, haven't we, Vic?' And he said, 'Sometimes.' And we laughed. We used to love to dance."

Patricia pointed to a little fairy on her collage. "I loved this mystical little fairy playing the violin and I put it in the middle because to me it referred to the dance that we had."

She pointed to more images: a couple dancing, entwined white swans forming a heart, wine, flowers, words such as "love," "family," and "friends." "These are all the good things that we've had in our life and I think we've been really blessed." She pointed to an image of a woman wrapping her arms around a man, "You know, my Vic still responds to a healing embrace. I think as caregivers, sometimes it feels like we are reaching for the impossible. There's a hopelessness

I feel, too, because no matter what we do he's not going to get better and I feel grief in all of this—nearly every day. The feeling of loss can be overwhelming, but I also need to cope with it and I think I do. Not only through prayer, but now allowing myself to remember the good times. I reflect on all that I am grateful for and I work on being positive." She chuckled as she said, "I also tell myself, 'what won't kill you will make you stronger.'" These words were also on her collage.

She said participating in the workshop was the impetus to get her focusing on what she felt mattered. It was her invitation to self-reflection and she found it to be therapeutic in terms of helping her cope with her grief and losses. "That day of the collage workshop, I stood looking at the Bristol board selection and I was thinking, do I want it white or do I want it black? I think every experience in life, even this sad time for me—there's still beauty in it. I chose the black because I just thought it looked nicer. It wasn't a macabre reason that I chose it." She laughed as she leaned into me and touched my arm, "I never want to be like everybody else, either, and everybody else was picking white. I just like being different, that's all."

I understood what she meant. Caregiving, like grieving, is unique. I found that when people were making their collages, they not only honored the person they were looking after, but also, and perhaps more importantly, recognized the reality of their losses, their grief, and the whole myriad of associated feelings. The participants were thoughtful and reflective through the experience. Once they selected a collection of images, it wasn't unusual for them to have a difficult time deciding what to include, what to leave out, what to put where, and what colors to use. I could see them not only making a collage but also working through their thoughts and feelings—some of which were right there on the surface, others much deeper and newly acknowledged. The collage-making workshops started out being about the product—how they represented their experience in images. However, the process turned out to be just as valuable as the product—perhaps even more so. For the participants, it was thought-provoking, sometimes emotional, and always enlightening to the point that some had realizations they were previously unaware of. For me, although I understood the value of creativity in one's life, regardless of the situation, I was struck by the degree of therapeutic benefit that participants received. I not only saw this through my own observations during the workshops but I also heard it commented on repeatedly by participants both during and after the workshops.

As I was listening to her story, I was moved by how eloquently she was able to put her thoughts to words. I was quiet as I pondered what she was saying while also looking at her collage, "Wow, thank you for sharing that, Patricia."

I asked Patricia if there was anything else that she wanted to tell me about her collage, or anything I hadn't asked about that she would like to share.

"Who is the audience that might be looking at these collages? What do you think they want to get out of them?"

"It will vary. Decision-makers, government officials, home care leaders, health care professionals at conferences, perhaps other caregivers. Those who read our articles and stories as well."

"I guess if anything, then, my message is to value what you've had. It's better to grow old and be inundated with good memories than to let the caregiving period of your life, with all its grief and the losses you experience, take all of the good memories away from you. It can happen if you allow it, but I'm not going to let it. Also, we're not the disease. I'm not defined by the diseases that I've had and neither is Vic. When others come to look after him, I want them to know he was a master electrician, a loving father, and a supportive loving husband. I don't want them to see some frail old man."

This was also something I heard often from caregivers. It was important to remember their loved one as they were before their illness, not how they were in sickness and various stages of frailty.

Patricia became a little teary as she continued, remembering a time when the police came after neighbors were worried when Vic went wandering. "I know the humiliation I've felt when police came to the door. I know that feeling of being washed up, not just for me as the caregiver but for Vic, too. It's horrible, I don't think anyone expects to deal with such grief while we are still living, but I don't know that anyone caused it. The police officers were absolutely adorable. They were so kind and so understanding. We needed that. It all helps. Kindness makes us feel like we still matter. We are here."

I had to smile. This was the first time I'd heard the police described as "adorable." I think age difference might have had something to do with it. The officers would have been much younger than Patricia and Vic, perhaps reminding her of her sons. But I think it mattered that they were compassionate, kind, and caring—qualities that are both immensely touching and important to caregivers.

"One thing I think about that makes me sad is that it's like a death in the family. It *is* a death in the family—only a slow one and we are anticipating what is to come nearly every day. Everybody reacts differently because everybody's relationship with that person has died and each one has been unique. Whether it's because you're the oldest child and your relationship with your dad was different than your younger brothers and sisters or things like that—we all handle grief in a different way and there's no right way and there's no wrong way. It's how you handle it. I don't think it's any different with caregivers. As a wife, I have a guy there that the kids dearly love as their dad. There's no question about that. He was a good father. He was my partner for all these years so my relationship with him was different from what the kids had but we all love him. We all want to do the right thing but there's always a difference in opinion on what the right thing is. If our son had his way, we would have the best that money could buy. But that's not important to me anymore. Are we grateful? Of course, we're grateful. But we were able to take the money from the sale of our house and just invest it. Our daughter's an angel, she's a nurse. I don't need to say much more but she's there every step of the way. We are going through it together, just differently."

I agreed. The grief experience and the process of working through it is as unique as each of us.

Myrna: My Mom

I heard various versions of what the caregivers I interviewed shared with me in my mother's words, "It's like I am married to a little old man. See how he sits in the car. He looks so small now." Or, I would hear, "I don't have a life partner anymore. He's not the man I married."

My mother would sometimes ask rhetorical questions: "Remember how solid and strong he was? Who would have thought this is how things would turn out?" She'd continue, "Your father! My God, Kimmie, he was the healthiest in his family. He was strong. Look at all of the physical work he did. He skated. There was no slowing him down. There was nothing he couldn't do. Now look at him."

When Mom said these things, all I could say was, "I know."

But I don't know. Not really. I don't know what it's like to lose your husband while he is still with you, to lose the social life you shared, to lose the person you talked to, confided in, laughed with, loved, every day. I don't know what it's like to lose the person who does practical things like fix whatever breaks down in the house, who ploughs and shovels the snow, or cuts the grass. I knew what it was like to lose my father, not my husband.

When I was growing up, Mom and Dad's life was active, vibrant, and loving. They went to dances with friends, hosted and went to parties. Dad went to his lodge meetings. As a Shriner he took part in many events and parades. He skated regularly—on racers—and often attended the old-time dance partner skating nights at the rink.

In the summer my parents would go to the steak dinner and dance every Wednesday at the CNR club in our community. He was active in the church, a member of the choir for as long as I can remember, and a church Elder. Dad started out in life as a fisherman like his father and brothers. After he left fishing, he continued with boat building with his brothers—big lobster boats. He was a Chief of the volunteer fire department for a time. Dad was vivacious and a highly engaged participant in life and community. He was happy.

So, I knew what it was like to lose my Dad, but I didn't know what it was like for my mother to lose her husband. Spousal caregivers rarely talk about their role as an intimate family caregiver without talking about the loss of their loved one, their life partner. The more I heard from spousal caregivers the closer I came to understand how much loss and grief affected them.

CHAPTER FOUR

Home Care and Other Services

"I think even talking about home care is a sore point of mine. I'm a very private person. The home care case manager was surprised that I was only asking for one hour. But I tell you very honestly, I was not looking forward to the person ringing the doorbell in the morning and sort of intruding into our lives. And that hour was," he stopped for a moment. *"It was enough."*
—Curtis

A Team Approach

FAMILY CAREGIVERS WORK WITH—AND negotiate around—all types of paid providers from the home care system, including health care aides, nurses, case managers, and rehabilitation professionals. Case managers are often the first professional in the home to complete the home care intake assessment and authorization for care. Both registered nurses (RNs) and licensed practical nurses (LPNs) can be engaged with the family caregiver for a variety to tasks including treatments such as wound care and patient teaching. Rehabilitation professionals assist with things like specialized equipment measuring and ordering, arranging for installation, or specialized rehab routines and exercises. Health care aides are the unregulated care providers who assist the client with personal care like bathing, feeding, and assistance with walking or toileting. Usually when someone needs home care it requires a cadre of people, all of whom do different things. At times, families can feel overwhelmed and frustrated, for as much as they appreciate what each professional offers, it sometimes seems like one doesn't know what the other is doing and they are receiving fragmented care. Their home feels more like a public institution rather than a private sanctuary.

Based on what I have come to know, we can do better. Care could be better coordinated and less intrusive with more regard for individual needs within the private space of someone's home. Regardless of how significant a role health care providers play in the life of a client and their family caregiver, that role is small when considered within the whole life of a family. Health care providers are only one cog in the wheel that the family caregiver needs to keep moving forward. Family caregivers' stories share what things work well for them and what parts of the system are failing them. As a researcher, I was excited to have such a rich source of data. As a health care professional, I was saddened at our occasional lack of compassion and support. We can do better.

Penny

I interviewed Penny at my university office a few years ago. An accountant who worked part-time so she could devote more time to her husband's care, she agreed to talk to me as part of a research study. When we met in a small interview room, the first thing she told me was how happy she was that I was doing this study, something all caregivers tell me in one way or another. "Boy oh boy," she said. "Do I have stories for you!"

I opened with a general question as I often do.

"Why don't we start by you telling me a little about your husband, how long you've been caring for him, and a bit about your life?"

Penny was very clinical in her response. Having done a lot of research on her own, she understood her husband's medical condition. She told me how Demetri developed nerve sensitivity nine years earlier. It started with some pain and it wasn't very long before he lost all sensation in the bottom of his feet and before long was experiencing severe neuropathy secondary to diabetes. They both attributed his symptoms and rapid deterioration to his diabetes.

Penny added, "Now it's attacking his autonomic system. And it's kind of interesting that I was the one who figured that one out from my research. I was with him at his doctor's appointment last September. Demetri has had difficulty swallowing for a few years now and the doctor had sent him for a test and he told us that the test had come back negative. I've since discovered that the test actually came back inconclusive because they had difficulty taking the blood, because of Demetri's condition. However, I said to the doctor last September, 'Do you think that the swallowing and esophagus problem is a result of the neuropathy attacking the autonomic system?' And he said, 'Yes, quite probably.' The doctor later told me it was an extremely bad case of neuropathy and, in fact, was the worst he'd encountered. It caused Demetri to be virtually immobile among a host of other issues."

Penny's knowledge of Demetri's condition and what might be happening with him is not unusual. Family caregivers are astute and intuitive when it comes to the care of their loved one. They not only provide care, but they also research conditions, determine opinions around the best course of action, and advocate for the best treatment.

"In February of this year, Demetri had an assessment with a geriatric doctor who said, 'Of course, it's the neuropathy that's now attacking the autonomic system,' and I thought, 'I could have told you that.'"

"Now, this is an extremely bad case of neuropathy. The doctor said it's the worst that he's ever seen. I imagine in some people, it only progresses to feeling sensation in a bit of the motor nerves. Demetri's condition deteriorated so much that now he's bedridden. He's totally immobile. He has great difficulty swallowing so getting pills and food into him is challenging. His esophagus seems to fill up very quickly because there's a problem with motility."

I leaned forward, observing Penny. She was businesslike and efficient with her conversation. Although her demeanor was professional, I noticed that her eyes teared up from time to time. She often wrung her hands in her lap.

"I kinda had to learn how to look after him as I've gone along. I'm an accountant." She added sarcastically, "You know, they didn't teach me this stuff in Accounting 101."

Demetri's neuropathy was advanced and it had attacked his motor nerves for the past three years. However, he did have a year of remission before the neuropathy came back and slowly spread to his major organs and bones. As Demetri's condition worsened, Penny was forced to reduce her work to part-time hours to continue caring for him. His mobility was poor and he would sit in his chair a good deal of the day. The couple had assistance from a paid provider—a health care aide—from the home care program each morning after Penny left for work. The instructions were always the same: be sure Demetri had water, a sandwich for his lunch, the television remote, and the phone in case he needed to call someone. The phone was especially important as Penny liked to call him every hour or so to check on him, and also to let him know when she would be home.

On occasion, the care provider would forget to leave the phone with Demetri. When that happened Penny panicked. "Was he choking? Did he fall? Is he unconscious? Does he need me?"

Her eyes watered and her voice quivered as she spoke those words.

She continued, "On those occasions I repeatedly called the house in the span of minutes. I couldn't concentrate on work. My frustration grew. Ultimately, I'd just leave work. Before I left, I reported to my supervisor and let them know that yet again, 'I need to leave early, I can't go to the meeting' and 'yes, I will take those files home and finish them tonight.' Inside, I'd be seething, frustrated, feeling inadequate as both an employee and as the wife I wanted to be."

Penny was animated as she spoke, using her arms to gesture as she recalled things. "I asked a lot of questions," she added. "I researched and I said to Demetri a few weeks ago, 'You're not getting the best care, but you're getting the best care I can give you.'"

Penny would arrive home, often not conscious of the route she drove, only to find her husband sitting in his chair absolutely fine. Demetri would always say, "Sorry, dear, the aide forgot to leave the phone with me today and I never noticed until she was gone." Feeling both relieved and angry, sometimes overcome with tears, she'd go into the kitchen and compose herself. There she would prepare for the second shift.

Penny said, "My first order of business was always to find out what happened on that particular day. I needed to know which care provider was here and why she didn't leave the phone. I would call the home care office for the supervisor. The last time I asked her who was supposed to be on the shift but," using air quotes, she continued, "'No, sorry.' She didn't know. I just hung up, annoyed that she didn't even offer to check for me. I was pretty sure it was a girl who was with Demetri and who had done this before."

I heard things like this many times. It is not necessarily one mistake or error in judgment that upsets family caregivers, but rather repetitious problems that lead them to believe that neither the caregiver nor the home care program cares enough to correct the issue.

It feels like blatant disregard for the family caregivers' wishes or compassion for their loved one.

Penny paused and let out a sigh before continuing.

"I couldn't let it go. An hour later I called the supervisor back, I wanted an answer and assurance that this would not happen again. Ever. I am getting so tired of the worry. I can't take the stress and I need to count on the care providers. We need consistency and reliability. When I reached the supervisor again, she assured me she tried to reach the aide on shift but she hadn't yet called her back. She promised me she would get me an answer but it would likely take a day. She just wasn't as concerned as I thought she should be. She even said, 'You know, your husband was alright, wasn't he? Did he cope okay without his phone?' Can you believe that? I just felt alienated; she didn't really understand why I was so upset and that just made me feel that there is no use in complaining. Nobody cares like I do."

When I ran our home care company, if an individual caregiver showed complete disregard for instruction to correct their behavior they would be reassigned and offered further education or, in some cases, be terminated. As well, supervisors were expected to follow up in a timely manner. All client phone calls had to be completed that day, even if it was to give the client or family caregiver an update that we were indeed following up on the problem. In my experience, family caregivers mostly want to know that supervisors are working hard to correct problems, that they are heard, and that their concerns are taken seriously. They need to be able to count on—and trust—those that are there to help them.

Reflecting on my research, it is the people who always come to mind first—the caregivers, the clients, their care aides, and nurses. It really is all about them. Everyone has a role to play and everyone needs to take responsibility for their part or things can go bad quickly. Health care is a system and there are processes for almost everything. One misstep is cause for concern.

Stories like Penny and Demetri's reinforced how far we need to come to support caregivers and clients through their caregiving journeys. As I listened to their accounts, I couldn't help reflecting on my personal situation—well, my parents' situation, actually. I remember how frustrated my mother, a retired RN, felt after some of her visits from her care aides, and even some nurses, when they didn't have the wherewithal, the expertise, or the compassion to be fully engaged in the home visit. When Mom felt listened to, she believed that people cared enough to remember and to follow through to give Dad the best possible care. That everyone was on top of things. When I interviewed caregivers, I was often reminded about how confidence in the home care nurse and other care providers means so much to families, almost everything really. Family caregivers need to be able to trust that others have the best interests of their loved ones at the top of their mind.

Expertise and competence are one thing, but compassion and empathy cannot be overlooked. In my experience, most care providers are competent but are sometimes not as conscientious when it comes to showing compassion and empathy. One doesn't need to be the team expert to make a difference for families. If the family caregiver and the client feel cared for and heard, their burden is eased.

The Assessment

When home care is called in to help, a case manager visits the client and family caregiver to determine their needs and what services could be offered. However, it is so standardized that sometimes a less-than-astute case manager might miss the opportunity to home in on unique family stressors. Another challenge is that home care is designed to meet the needs of the client only, not the family caregiver or anyone else who might be in the home. This can be problematic, particularly when the family caregiver is ill or has multiple demands such as a job, community roles, or young children. Assessments are becoming more comprehensive in that caregiver burden, strengths, and gaps are often assessed, but rarely are services allocated that address the needs of the caregiver—some of which could strengthen their resilience.

While in most cases the family caregiver is present for the assessment, their needs are often overlooked. Comprehensive components of the client situation are addressed, including their physical status, functional ability in terms of bathing, dressing, eating, mobility, their support—which is where the family caregiver comes in, as well as resources the family may already have in place or that may also help, such as meal programs or transportation—and often a full physical assessment on the client is done. It is also common to do a safety assessment to see if there are risks to the client such as scatter rugs that could cause a fall. An environmental assessment is part of the overall assessment to ensure a safe environment for staff to provide care, such as bed height if care is done in the bed, outside lighting, whether or not it is a smoking environment, the presence of pets, and anything else that might affect the health and safety of care providers. Although currently some tools to assess the family caregiver burden or impact of caregiving are beginning to be used in some jurisdictions, they are often data collection tools with little in the way of resources added to the service plan.

Carol and Todd told me about their assessment experience. They both felt one thing that was missed was sit down with them, either separately or together, and ask, "Now, what impact is this having on you? Can we assist with anything? Is there anything you'd like to talk about?" There was no inquiry about their ability to keep doing what they were doing. They believed that in situations like theirs, where intense daily care and monitoring was required to properly care for Max, the caregivers alone should have been asked in a separate conversation, "What's the biggest problem on your plate right now?"

Todd felt they could have been flourishing much better rather than floundering.

Todd felt they should have asked Carol specifically, as he was still going about his normal life. He was maintaining his full-time work and was in and out of the house as usual. He participated in most of his outside activities. He said he was used to looking after basic household chores by that point—cutting the grass, shoveling snow, and attending to anything that needed fixing—and felt that was his role. But beyond that, as far as the actual caregiving and what was going on with Carol, she was handling it all.

The notion of flourish versus flounder needs more attention in caregiving. Unfortunately, all too often we accept floundering as okay. I remember one early research study in which a case manager actually told me we put in just enough services to keep them coping. "If they aren't falling apart then we have to be okay with that. There just aren't enough resources." This is not okay. It is not acceptable and inhumane. The feeling that we're hardly able to cope, exhausted, not doing enough, or not being enough affects our ability to be resilient. Family caregivers feel like they are barely able to keep their heads above water because the system is seemingly set up to keep them there.

Donelle

Donelle was the first caregiver I interviewed through my research studies; I remember her well. Donelle was particularly articulate about providing care to her husband and dealing with the health care system, most likely because she herself was a retired pharmacist who often worked with home care clients and family caregivers. Her pharmacist role came across to me as important to her sense of self. It shaped her identity, as well as the expectations she had of herself in her role as her husband's caregiver.

My most poignant recollection of Donelle's story was the fierce lack of empathy she experienced among the home care nurses on their case. Donelle said they seemed to lack the ability to just talk to her husband as they assessed his pain and other symptoms. She described their use of the pain scale—rating pain on a scale of one to ten where ten is the worse pain possible—as a barrier to their full engagement with her husband. She recalled one nurse who stood out as amazing. Her husband loved it when she came to see him. I asked her why.

"Because she would talk to him. She would assess him throughout the conversation during her visit. She was clearly an expert. She didn't have to pull out the ruler to show him the numbers or the smiley faces and ask him to point to where he was on the scale today or rate his pain on a scale from one to ten."

Donelle appreciated the way this particular nurse was intuitive and proficient.

She continued, "She *talked* to him, she *touched* him, she *looked* at him, she *engaged* with him. She could tell how he was feeling by watching his facial expressions, the way he grimaced when he moved, and what he described throughout the conversation. She made him feel that this visit was as important to her as it was to him. That was a good thing. She would of course verify her observations with him before she left, but she gave us holistic care. Neither of us felt as if things were missed or left unsaid after her visit."

More than others, Donelle described home care as a thorn in her side. I think of her experience almost as an "in spite of" situation. That is, her husband stayed home *in spite of* home care, not because of it. Donelle described situations where she felt frustrated, annoyed, or exhausted—and she was particularly annoyed with the "on a scale of one to ten tell me about your pain" comments which, she said, drove her nuts.

"I also had to fight and martial my own resources for the midazolam drip. I was made to feel that I wanted euthanasia for my husband! Many times I was frustrated. The care I *was* offered from home care was actually unhelpful because a PCA [paid unregulated care provider] wasn't going to solve my problems. Although, I need to admit as hard as it was, and as stressful as it was, it was still better for me than nothing."

Donelle felt her negative experiences were a reflection of poor policy implementation, procedures, and guidelines, rather than bad people. She said, "They were trying to follow protocol and procedure, like the one-to-ten pain scale. What they did didn't work for me always or even often. I had needs that weren't being met. In terms of the support that they did provide, once I found the right support, incredible. It was just hard."

Donelle felt it would have been more helpful had she known what services were available to her. A better understanding of what was possible would have enabled her to know what would have worked well for them, rather than to have things provided that didn't quite work—such as the health care aide at night who wasn't able to give medications. Donelle felt that if home care spent more time educating her on home care and the various kinds of services they offered at the outset—before any services were even put in the home—some of the problems would have been avoided. This would have saved home care time and money and spared her unnecessary frustration.

Donelle was her husband's rock. She had to be. He was failing—nightly. Her crystal-clear vision of what constituted good care guided everything she did for him day in and day out. That was her guide post and she expected her husband should receive excellent care from outside help as well. To point this out to the case manager and nurses would require her to be clear with her words and brilliant with her approach. Her education as a pharmacist gave her insider wisdom, a knowing that she could get her point across clearly while keeping their relationship with their health care team intact. She let go of some services like the health care aides at night and called on some of her friends. She shifted the hours home care offered between day and night-time. She asked for LPNs after learning that she could indeed be assigned nurses for medication administration.

Once Donelle figured out more of the system, she molded what was happening with home care until she was satisfied. She observed early on what was creating many of the problems—too little time, a poorly resourced program, ill-prepared case managers, and although she hated to think it, a fundamental lack of compassion.

She felt that some of the people working for home care just didn't seem well conditioned to deal with cases like theirs. She remembered the discomfort she felt when some friends and extended family members would ask how she was doing as the main caregiver for her husband. She got the strong impression many times that no one really wanted to hear what she had to say. "I wanted to scream at them, 'Please do not hold the god damn door knob and ask me, 'How are you feeling, Donelle?'"

Family caregivers want health care providers to take the time to be engaged and relaxed while they are doing a home visit. They deserve fulsome time and attention from health care providers. Time that is focused on them with a genuine interest in doing a thorough assessment into how things are going, giving the client and family caregiver time to fully explain what is going well, what is worrisome, and what might be falling apart. But it can be difficult for family caregivers to think on their feet. If they feel the nurse or case manager is rushed—which unfortunately is common—then they won't open up. "Why bother?" is a natural reaction.

Falling into the "why bother" trap can be self-depreciating and self-destructive. Such feelings can fester and grow allowed. In my experience, when caregivers say nothing as they watch their case manager leave the home or feel rushed out of their physician's office, they often feel defeated and it can be paralyzing. This is often the time caregivers need to dig deep within themselves and muster both courage and energy to speak up and stand firm.

Reminders When you Feel Defeated or Think "Why Bother?"

- Do not apologize.
- Do not undervalue what you do and what you believe.
- Taking action is not about pleasing others.
- Ask yourself, "What do I truly want from this encounter?"
- Don't settle.
- You have the right to be heard and to ask questions.

Positive thoughts, or self-talk, can be empowering and help family caregivers stay in control of a situation that they have the right to manage.

It was stories like Donelle's that told me we have a long way to go to support caregivers and clients on home care. When caregivers feel listened to and valued, they have more confidence in their home care team. When they are given time to fully express their concerns, they are better able to ask pertinent questions to ensure they understand what is being said. This can instill confidence in the caregiver, who then feels that nurses and case managers will follow up and follow through on what's needed. Confidence in the individual home care nurses means so much to families—almost everything, really.

Confidence can be instilled when health care providers demonstrate compassion, empathy, and caring. When these are lacking, family caregivers assume they don't care. The natural progression of thinking is that if they don't care then they aren't going to act on requests, they aren't going to be proactive in offering resources, and they aren't capable of meeting the family caregiver and client needs.

While competence is important, and most nurses *are* competent, they don't need to be the team expert to make a difference and be a great home care nurse in the eyes of the family caregiver. If a caregiver and the client feel cared for and about, and if they feel heard, their burden is eased, they take comfort, and they can believe in their ability to be in charge of the care of their loved one.

I noted a contradiction in what Donelle was telling me. At one point she claimed that "I don't think I could have had that support from home care." But she follows it up a few minutes later by saying, in a slightly different context, "In terms of the support they provide, incredible." I have heard these ambiguities before—exemplary care or care that was lacking, confidence in care providers or concern they weren't doing their job, feeling the benefit of home care or feeling the burden of home care. These feelings, seemingly at odds with one another, arise because, although outside services often fall short of a family's expectations, the client still appreciates any help that eases their burden even a little.

It is also a self-fulfilling prophecy. If family caregivers believe people, like their case manager and other health care professionals, are competent and compassionate, then they have confidence that the system will be there for them. If family caregivers perceive they have a support system, including home care, that they can count on, then they can achieve a greater sense of self-efficacy. That is, they believe they can be a good, if not great, caregiver for their loved one, or at least that they have the skills to figure out how to continue moving forward in a positive way. It gives them the courage to keep on going.

Carol and Todd

Carol and Todd had a lot to say about their home care experience.

"We had home care for over a year and a half," Carol said. "We received three hours once a week."

Todd added, "It just allowed Carol and I to get out on a Wednesday afternoon. It was the advantage, a fact that one of us could be away and doing things and the other one would be here. But still, there are times when you just want to get out together."

Even though they felt as if they were racing against time, having a care aide sit with Max every Wednesday did give Carol and Todd peace of mind—something in short supply for caregivers.

"It was a relief," Carol said.

"Very much so," agreed Todd. "Far more, in fact, for Carol than on me. And that's where most of the impact occurs, in a situation where it's husband and wife that are looking after, it falls on the wife. There is absolutely no question about that."

Carol nodded, "We've seen that happen time and time again with other acquaintances in the same situation. There's no doubt that the male partner does a fair amount of work, but the burden of the day-to-day care tends to fall on the woman, I think."

Todd emphasized, "Not *think*, *know*." He laughed, "It's not a *think*."

I knew what Todd was getting at. Women are most often the primary caregiver within families. They often bear most of the responsibility for childcare and then later in life for their parents, in-laws, or aging friends or relatives. However, this disproportionate ratio is gradually shifting and now as many as 40% of caregivers in the United States are men and as many as 46% in Canada. However, there continues to be diversity in the type of tasks and number of hours that men and women contribute. There is more awareness of the gendered nature of caregiving, and just as more dual-parent families are both in the workforce, men and women are increasingly sharing childcare as well as eldercare responsibilities.

This was the case with Carol and Todd, and I could tell they were in sync by the way they told me their story. They saw their caregiving responsibilities in partnership, a luxury not afforded to many family caregivers. They talked about how they naturally took on various caregiving assignments depending on things like their mutual work schedules and the tasks each of them were more adept or comfortable with. For example, Carol was a natural organizer. A freelance writer, she was used to organizing her time to get everything done. She was a proficient multi-tasker and used to keeping many activities going at the same time. Todd maintained the house and heavier tasks as he had in their previous home. He was the main chauffeur for Max as well—driving him to his lodge meetings, to coffee with friends, or simply getting out to give Carol time to catch up with things at home. Arranging for respite once a week gave them a break.

"Were you the one who initiated getting respite services from home care?" I asked Todd.

Carol jumped in, "No. I did."

"And was there any resistance on the part of your father-in-law?" I asked.

Carol replied, "No, because he was still relatively sharp and he realized that I needed a break and he knew it wasn't a bad thing."

Todd chimed in, "Dad appreciated what Carol was doing, there's no question about that, and he made it known to his friends and acquaintances in no uncertain terms. But I think he realized the fact that at the time, Carol was just gradually wearing down and something had to change."

The burnout and other effects of caregiving are not always obvious and often appear gradually. A spouse or close friend or relative is usually the first to notice that family caregivers are suffering from stress, fatigue, or even exhaustion. When this happens, it may be because their sleep may be interrupted by the one being cared for, or there are just too many things to get done in a day so the caregiver foregoes sleep to get everything done. They could also be experiencing insomnia due to the stress of caregiving and the nature of what they are coping with. Other signs that caregiving is affecting them in a negative way may be weight loss or weight gain due to poor nutrition and a lack of physical activity, bowel problems, or even hair falling out. There are myriad symptoms that can be caused by the stress of caregiving and the effects can be as individual as the caregiver.

Todd carried on, "There's no doubt that there are stressors when you move into somebody's home. Now it might be different if, let's say, this had been our home and my father had moved in with us— totally different situation. In this case, this was his home. He was used to a certain pattern of activity and we maintained that as much as possible. In fact, I'd say, very much so. But stepping into family caregiving and getting home care affects everyone's privacy and," Max paused, "it affects your freedom."

I know what he meant. I remembered going home to visit Mom and Dad during the years we had home care and respite, whether I was on my own, with my husband and son, or all of us siblings were there for a big family get together. It felt like a disruption in the natural order of things. We never felt comfortable sleeping in and lounging about over coffee as things needed to be done, like getting our showers, making breakfast, tidying up, or getting laundry started. Home care came at 8:00 every morning and it affected our routine. We made sure to help Mom do what she did before they came—empty the catheter bag, wash Dad's hands and face, get him ready for breakfast, and sometimes feed him—and then worked our time around the bathroom to not interrupt their schedule with Dad.

We had a large four-bedroom home with one bathroom. As kids, we were used to hurrying, sharing, and multiple people needing their time to shower and get ready for the day. We all had to be ready for the school bus at 7:40, Dad made our breakfast as Mom was off to work by 5:30. Dad left for work right after the school bus left. Most mornings there were two or three of us in the bathroom at the same time—whether it was at the sink brushing teeth, in the mirror curling hair, or even someone on the toilet or in the shower—we were used to sharing and doubling up. Now, with home care arriving each morning, things seemed even more rushed.

On respite days, every Tuesday and Friday, we all left for town so Mom could keep her routine. You might wonder why we didn't cancel with all of us home for a week or two, but Mom didn't want to interrupt the schedule of the care providers she had grown to know and wanted to keep. To change things could risk not getting the same care providers back. There were also various errands to be done on those days—grocery and any other shopping, paying bills, appointments, or picking up library books. We all jumped in to help with various things for both Mom and Dad, but messing with the home care schedules and routines was not feasible. Many families feel the same way, particularly when they find people and routines that work well. So, we got used to giving up our privacy from eight to ten most mornings and going out each Tuesday and Friday from eight until noon. It was a nuisance but we grew to accept it.

Carol explains, "One of the other issues with home care was the fact that I just got that three-hour break. The one time when we did go away to a conference, it wasn't easy. We'd made arrangements for home care to come in and check on him, to make sure he had his lunch. One of our neighbors happily volunteered to come in, too, so they popped in from time to time. Apparently, the care provider missed a day. I was concerned because I don't think Dad had his meds properly that day. When we had a word with the visiting nurse, his case manager I believe it was, she said that she didn't realize there was a missed shift. Dad's mental faculties would go up and down depending on his blood work and what we didn't realize was that he was about to head into another bout of anemia. So, he was pretty fuzzy and we really didn't get any kind of support for that. I just had to provide more of the care and be more diligent myself. We still could only get the approved respite and nobody seemed to check whether or not the worker was here or not. If it wasn't for the neighbor checking, we would not have known. I was extremely disappointed with that."

That's one of the risks that sometimes happens with home care. If the family caregiver is home, they will report a no show. However, a client who has mild confusion or a type of dementia may not realize the caregiver didn't show up. They have no means to contact the home care office or service provider agency when there's a no show. No shows can happen for a variety of reasons—a car accident, an unreported illness by the caregiver, or lateness if they are running behind with another client. Most service provider organizations have extensive policies, procedures, and standards that all staff must abide by. Staff are expected to call into the office any time they need replacement or if they are going to be late so the client and family can be notified, but they may not, which is when the system breaks down. As much as families are told to call in if the caregiver is late or a no show, if the client is struggling with confusion, the office doesn't get notified to send a replacement.

That was one of the most difficult things I had to deal with in owning a service provider agency for twenty-five years. I found nothing as frustrating as when the health care aide or nurse did not give the level of care I expected and according to policies—including not calling in if they were sick or running late. Although it is a rare occurrence considering the thousands of visits a large organization does each month, if you are the client expecting someone and they do not show up it is a big problem, and to me completely unacceptable. If it happens more than once it is usually grounds for dismissal as it leaves clients and families at risk.

Carol and Todd worked and had responsibilities outside the home and at times left home a short time before the caregiver was due to arrive. Family caregivers rely on home care to show up. If family caregivers are out of town for respite or some other reason, as Carol and Todd were, things can fall apart and as much as family caregivers put a schedule in place it might not go as planned. Whether it was a mix up in the care providers' schedule, car trouble, or a sick call, it is important that home care or the service provider agency be notified so they can act on it and send a replacement or find out where the expected caregiver is. They can't intervene if they don't know about it. It is one of the things that is difficult for family caregivers and there needs to be safeguards in place to avoid or minimize missed shifts without notice. Families could have an arrangement with the organization to call the home when the caregiver is due to arrive, or better, have the family caregiver or another relative check in on each expected visit. It is impossible to predict unforeseen circumstances and that is often the reason for most missed visits or lateness. It is one of the inherent risks with home care that isn't present when someone is in care in a facility.

Todd reminded her, "You were furious, never mind disappointed."

Carol said, "Well, I was furious that they didn't come in."

Todd continued, "It could have resulted in a serious situation. Fortunately, it didn't and that's a positive."

Carol continued, "And it didn't, but that meant that basically for a little bit more than two years, I got three hours off a week with the exception of that one weekend."

Although Carol and Todd played different caregiving roles, they were a solid team and a great support to one another. I don't always see this kind of support for the main family caregiver. There can be conflicts among family members or situations where one doesn't like what the other is doing; for example, if one sibling thinks a parent is safe in the home and the others don't and want their parent in a care facility.

I most often see conflict when the people who might be best to support the family caregiver either don't live in the same town or don't take an active role in the well-being of either the family caregiver or the one being cared for. They come in and out of their lives, thinking they can problem solve or make a workable, but far from perfect, situation better. Some of it boils down to family dynamics; however, these are often more pronounced when everyone is worried about an ill parent. In home care, we sometimes call this the "California Daughter Syndrome." Nothing against California, but the notion is that other family members parachute in—with the best of intentions—and get involved in decision-making without fully understanding the reality of the daily caregiving grind. I can recall situations where a family member intervened with care as soon as they got to town. They would call home care to complain about what was in place or demand different services—sometimes without the knowledge of the primary caregiver. At that point home care, as well as the service provider organization, becomes entangled in family dynamics. It is outside of the responsibility of home care to sort through these dynamics, but they still get caught in the middle as they try to keep everyone at ease. This is one of the main reasons why home care requires only one or two contacts to coordinate services—the family dynamics are left with the family to sort out. With Todd and Carol, they were in sync from the beginning.

I clarified, "It sounds like that weekend might have broken your trust with the system?"

Todd said, "It did, yeah."

The biggest issue family caregivers have with outside care is finding services and workers they can trust. Families need to know that workers can be trusted to show up on time every time. They need to feel that this person can be trusted to do the job, and trust that things will happen as planned and agreed to. When people let family caregivers down—even once—that trust is broken, and it takes longer to regain it every time it is lost.

Perhaps because I've seen what a breach of trust can do to families—both in working with so many over my years in home care, and also through witnessing it in my own family—I firmly believe it is only the family caregiver and client who get to claim whether trust is there or not. It is one thing for the family caregiver to trust home care or the service provider organization in general; it is something else for the family caregiver to trust the care providers who are present in their home and providing hands-on care to their loved one. It is the care provider themself that needs to work to instill trust with the families they work with.

Care providers earn trust and keep it by following the plan of care as set out with the case manager and family caregiver, by showing up on time every time, by demonstrating care and compassion for the one they are caring for, by being friendly and engaging with the family caregiver, and by providing safe and competent care. If trust is not there, it can lead to a revolving door of care providers or nurses to get to a place where the family trusts all of the people coming to provide care.

Carol continued, "I felt I couldn't trust them to be there for us. And I don't think it's reasonable to expect somebody—us—to be on call, giving full-time care twenty-four hours a day, seven days a week for the duration of someone's life. And that's what it was. It wasn't so much the nursing care and other things I did, but the fact that for a lot of the time you're constantly in a state of hypervigilance, especially with conditions like I've described. The health of the person you're caring for goes up and down and up and down."

She paused. Todd looked as if he were collecting his thoughts to add something more. "I know I'm going around the same bush again," Todd said. "I go back to those two items of privacy and freedom. I think in a lot of cases where you get seniors, they're used to spending a lot of their time with each other so it doesn't impact as much on paper but I think it impacts psychologically on the caregiver. Just to be able to get out, whether it's to go and do shopping or whether it's just to walk down the road, or if the old boy wants to go to the pub and have a beer. Which you can't do."

They were talking about the effect of being so involved with the health system—everyone telling them what they should do or not do—and either feeling judged or feeling pushed to advocate harder for their loved one. They felt judged that they weren't doing enough— taking deserved time for themselves, asking for additional respite hours, leaving Max on his own for a few hours, even though that was safe. Through it all, they were sometimes exhausted and always doing the best they could. They felt judged that what they were doing was somehow substandard, yet there was no offer for more help which led them to advocate more and to be more aggressive than they felt necessary to get more care or a different kind of care. Many caregivers feel like Todd and Carol. Most want to be able to have a conversation and express what they are dealing with and what they need. Most prefer to do it without becoming angry or feeling that they are being too demanding, both of which perpetuate the family caregivers' stress level and mental anguish over trying to do the best for their loved one.

Carol added, "I remember getting a prescription. Sometimes Max had difficulty sleeping so we found a mild anti-anxiety drug and prescribed it off label. Its principal side effect was drowsiness. By the time you've taken enough to quell your anxiety, you're out cold. But normally Max would prefer a shot of scotch before he's going to bed. So, I get a young pharmacist and he says, 'You haven't refilled this for a while.' I said, 'Yes, he's been having a shot of scotch before he goes to bed.' He says, 'Well, he shouldn't be drinking.' I said, 'He's eighty-six-years-old. If he wants a drink in his own house before he goes to bed, he's going to have a drink. But the important thing is that he has a drink a day to balance the blood thinners.' The pharmacist says, 'Oh but, you know, do you really think he should?' I said, 'At least let the man have it.'"

Todd added, "Something to look forward to."

Just as family caregivers know what their loved ones need to live a safe and comfortable life, family caregivers themselves also deserve a good quality of life. Although family caregivers know what might help them maintain their own health and happiness, many don't feel they have access to the things to support them in doing that—the things that will sustain them and their ability to care for their loved one. Things like appropriate home care from people they trust; sufficient respite—tailored to their needs rather than a one-size-fits-all approach; time to ask trusted health care professionals' opinions; access to information, equipment, and supplies in a timely manner; respect; and to be valued for their contributions in the care and support of their loved one.

I remember one visit home, five or six years before Dad died. It was a time when he had so many daily requirements, such as bathing and dressing, preparing food and feeding, emptying his catheter, and getting him into his mechanical lift. This care was provided by Mom and his home care aides from the local home care program. The aides were good, but they weren't proactive enough in their care or problem solving to fully meet Dad's needs. It wasn't that his paid workers had poor skills or didn't care, but as Dad's disease progressed the level of help he required also progressed, and even small incremental changes made a huge difference. For example, fatigue caused him to choke more than usual when eating or drinking which could make the difference between choking or not. A developing urinary tract infection could cause him to go from being alert and communicative to having less strength, sleeping more, and being so dull as to appear almost unresponsive. The paid care providers had basic skills that could meet the needs of most of their clients, but their time was limited and they were highly task focused—they adhered to a care plan or a list of duties that were often built to fill the time allocated, whether it was fifteen minutes for a medication or twenty minutes to feed him. There was no room for deviation from the care plan and Dad's condition fluctuated daily, as is common with people living with chronic or life-limiting conditions. Dad's need for nuanced care couldn't be met by short visits and a specific list of tasks, so it meant that Mom had to pick up the slack. She was action-oriented and did what needed to be done. The loving, intuitive care Mom gave Dad was because she was his wife, not because she was a former maternity nurse.

Mom knew how to feed him without choking him. She knew how to tell if his urine was becoming concentrated, which prompted her to give him more fluids so he wouldn't become dehydrated. There are so many things that I saw her do that were anticipatory and proactive in his care. Those were the things that kept him well.

Patricia

Patricia, who cared for her husband for five years before he died after complications due to dementia, said, "If you want us to keep our loved ones in our homes, give us the support we need to do it. I think we're going in the right direction, I just think that the direction needs to be refined a bit. Just like they say dementia is a big umbrella with fifty some spokes in it, the analogy also works in caregiving where there are also many spokes."

Patricia was referring to workshops offered to caregivers dealing with dementia. Alzheimer's is the disease that most commonly comes to mind, but dementia is actually an umbrella term for many diseases affecting memory, cognition, and reasoning. It's a growing concern around the world, both in terms of the disease itself and the demands it places on caregivers of people with dementia and the communities in which they live. Globally, initiatives are increasing with regard to how we care for people with dementia, and in building dementia-friendly communities. In communities around North America, there are workshops for caregivers and community members to support understanding the disease, its proliferation, and effects, and also offering strategies on caregiving and using outside services like home care.

Catastrophic and life-limiting conditions like dementia, multiple sclerosis, amyotrophic lateral sclerosis, rheumatoid arthritis, other chronic and autoimmune disorders as well as end-of-life care are all a tremendous societal concern that require extensive home care and also escalate the needs of caregivers. Patricia's use of a large umbrella is effective when thinking of the family caregiver and the many facets needed to support them.

She continued, "We need a hub—someone in the middle of it to direct caregivers to all the spokes they need or need to know about. Maybe home care isn't always the right avenue. Maybe they need to be directed here or there," she pointed with her finger, "but it seems right now that I'm the hub. I am the one that's doing it all, finding everything out on my own, and pushing for what we need."

I asked, "Is your case manager directing you to some resources as well?

Patricia said, "Well, I liked her well enough but it was trial and error. It isn't like I didn't think she cared or that she didn't want what was best for us. I just didn't feel that she was the hub of the group. She didn't act that way. In retrospect, I think she should have. It would have saved me a lot of energy. I had to advocate for everything, when in actuality it was all out there and available, but it wasn't offered."

Patricia illustrated a conflict she experienced in her care. "Home care says that case managers are the hub, the coordinator of the care, the go-to for us but they certainly weren't in our case." The case manager is the one who coordinates the care and helps with equipment needs to make care easier. They know where the community resources are—support groups, meal support, day programs for clients with various conditions, medical supplies at good prices—or they should. They are in the best position to be that hub. Given that most home care programs position the case manager as the first point of contact and the resource for the client and family as part of their role and responsibility, it is reasonable for the client to expect them to take on that role. So when the case manager doesn't follow through on that part of their role, care and support for both the client and family caregiver falls between the cracks leading to poor coordination and a lack of services and supports that could help. The family caregiver becomes their own advocate with no one following through to ensure they have what they need. The outcome is variable depending on how well the family caregiver can advocate; in some cases, inadequate care and support is the result.

A Guide to Getting the Services You Need

Advocating for yourself or your loved one simply means asking for what you need. But you need to know how to ask for something and where to seek support.

Be open and honest about what you need and have your reasons prepared. Here are a few things to keep in mind when you're looking for information, care, and services:

Where to look?
- Caregiver associations have dedicated staff to provide support, information, advocacy, and navigation for caregivers.
- Disease- and disability specific organizations focus on the needs of clients with specific conditions like the MS society, Parkinson's society, spinal cord injury associations, cerebral palsy association. Sometimes these organizations have supports specifically for caregivers of people with various conditions.
- Seniors organizations. With many older people becoming caregivers, seniors' centers often have programs, referral and information services, or services for caregivers.

(Continued)

- Health Department information line. This might be an 811 or 211 service in your area. Here is where to look for social workers, case managers, or home care. You can call the information line to get numbers for home care or other programs in your area. Home care is the department that does assessments to determine your eligibility for care in your home.
- For crisis support, call a distress or crisis line. They are often a source of support and know where to direct you depending on your need. Many have a directory for various community services and supports.
- Financial benefits supports are available to caregivers depending on eligibility; your area may have a benefit center through your local state or provincial government.

When you need help with information or advocacy, many of the places listed above have people designated as caregiver advisors or system navigators. If this service is not offered to you, ask if they have such a person.

How to ask?
- Regardless of how you ask for something, keep a written record for yourself. Document the date, who you talked to or left a message with, what your request was, and the result.
- Do you need to follow up? If they say they will follow up with you, ask for a due date and let them know that you will follow up shortly after that date if you haven't received any feedback or action.
- You may feel like a nuisance, but this can save you steps later if you don't get what you need right away. A paper trail can help you get action if your request goes unanswered for days or weeks on end. Having accurate information at your fingertips will let others know you are organized,

competent, and determined to get your needs met. It is harder to defer someone who is ready with detailed information than someone who can't recall details such as who they last talked to, when, and the details of the conversation.

- Be direct, clear, and polite. Be open about what you need and why. Although it is not your problem, many of the people you will be seeking out are busy and possibly overworked. While they should be there for you, the client or the customer, in reality they likely have multiple people they are talking to and assisting, so make things easy for them.

- Most of us want to work with people who are kind, so don't underestimate politeness regardless of what you get back in return. If someone isn't helpful, you can bring your request to their supervisor if needed, but first try your best to get what you need on your first call.

- For home care, your case manager is usually your main contact and should be in a position to help you get the care you need. If you do not feel heard despite repeated requests, then it is time to take things further. Their supervisor, who might be a team leader or the director of the home care program, is your next stop. If you don't feel comfortable approaching them, then organizations that support caregivers can help. Places like caregiver associations, eldercare, or even a patient advocate might exist within your area.

Lavonne

"I just wish they would please take more time to talk to us family caregivers when they come in. Not to just like," Lavonne snapped her fingers, "in and out."

I asked, "Is this your message to all health care providers, not only case managers?"

"I find that the doctor's appointments are," she paused, "a little brief—because we had it better in the past and when you get spoiled then you miss it, right?"

She was referring to the fairly recent past when physicians weren't so rushed. I hear from many caregivers, as well as friends and colleagues, that physicians are limiting the time they spend with their patients at an appointment, often confining the discussion to one medical complaint. This is not conducive to comprehensive, compassionate care, yet with the aging population and the growth in the number of people with multiple chronic and sometimes acute conditions, physicians believe it is the only way they can get through their day.

I could hear both frustration and fatigue in Lavonne's voice and that saddened me. It's disheartening to hear first-hand experiences illustrating that our health care services do seem to be in a state of decline. We are clearly not meeting people's needs.

I asked, "Did you have a doctor that took longer with you and gave you more of what you needed?"

She continued, "Yes. Good Lord, and now if we go see him... he'll say, 'Besides that, how are things going?' and go on and on without really hearing me. So I feel like we are just shoved out the door, you know? And the caregiving," she said, referring to care providers coming into her home. "Well, I hope I'm not going to need people to come in, but eventually, you know, when it does come to that, I think I'd prefer to have somebody stay with us. I would rather that than put my husband in a home. I go there to visit other people and I find that it's a good place for some, but a lot of people, like my friends and other family, they worry when their loved one is there. You just don't know what happens when you're not there."

I nodded and waited for her to continue.

"The affordability of medical equipment and supplies is another thing. My husband was diagnosed six years ago but I think he had Parkinson's way before that. I remember going to his appointments and we asked to get a parking pass or something because he does have trouble walking but also getting out of the vehicle—the spots are so small. It wasn't that he couldn't walk but getting out of the car in a regular stall was hard."

I clarified, "oh, you are referring to a parking pass for someone with disabilities?"

She nodded and continued, "so that was okay and I think in this country we're really quite lucky. I don't know about having home care come to our house yet, but the one thing that I hope I won't have trouble with this coming winter is DATS [transportation for people with disabilities]. I will not be driving myself to the Parkinson's clinic so I hope to be able to get DATS. Apparently, that's not easy and that is a big concern for me."

DATS services are a necessity for many and well-used in many jurisdictions, so the wait-times can be longer for a few reasons—weather, the varying abilities of riders, and sometimes over-booked schedules. Although many caregivers rely on this service, it can bring challenges, such as making extra time for pick-ups and drop-offs to appointments, and ensuring someone is waiting with the client as they can be at risk if the driver is late or in some cases misses the pick-up and needs to be called.

Lavonne continued, "Before, for other things, I had them tell me he doesn't qualify because of this and that. When he couldn't work anymore a few years ago and he wasn't yet sixty-five. I phoned Aids to Daily Living [a program that provides some medical equipment and supplies for those who qualify] and I said, we really can't afford all these Depends and stuff. I don't know how many times I called. I said he goes through two or three of the max size pads and a diaper a day, and they are very expensive. They told me, 'Oh, that's not enough, you won't qualify.' Well," Lavonne paused and shook her head, "they said because he doesn't change it every hour he won't qualify. That is ridiculous because I could change it out every hour, but we conserve."

There are no rewards for being frugal and responsible with products and services which would ultimately save government money. We reward the wrong things, like overuse.

Lavonne added, "There could be much better support and costs covered for those kinds of products. So many people need them and it is only going to get worse. Apart from that, I haven't got really any complaints as of yet because I haven't had to use many other services. I do it all. He wants me to."

I often hear that the spouse who is being cared for wants their husband or wife to do all of the caregiving. And for the most part, the spouse wants to provide that care. While spouses typically want to care for each other and get satisfaction in being able to care for each other there are additional stressors. In addition to financial burdens and the lack of recognition for being responsible with resources, spouses experience more physical effects that affect caregiver health, as well as social and mental impacts because their relationship drastically changes, and their social life diminishes leading to more loneliness, alienation from friends, and even depression.

One of the benefits of spousal caregiving is that they live together, so there is usually someone in the home more often than if the caregiver lived away from their loved one. But they also need better caregiver supports and resources. The rules and criteria don't always make sense. In this case, if it weren't a spouse conscious of resources, and more paid help had to come into the home, they may have been less judicious with supplies and used more. Caregivers then begin to think, why bother? Being frugal and resourceful can sometimes leave them worse off.

Curtis

Curtis, an eight-two-year-old widower, cared for his wife following a series of severe strokes. He really wanted to share his story. Widowed for a few years by the time I met him, Curtis welcomed me to his home, a tidy, well-kept bungalow. I got the impression from my surroundings that they hadn't changed much since Mary had died. There were lots of knick-knacks on the bookshelves and entertainment stand. As well, there were doilies on most surfaces and cloths covering the armrests of the sofa and chairs—things that I haven't generally noticed in homes where men have been living alone for a number of years.

Curtis told me he enjoyed writing. In fact, he had captured most of what they lived through in a manuscript that he wrote. He shared it with me in the hopes that it would be useful. Throughout the interview, he would give a head nod toward the pages on the coffee table between us and tell me, "It's all in there."

While I knew that much of their journey included long hospital stays as well as a time in long-term care, my first question was related to the care they received at home. I asked Curtis if he had any idea of what home care would be or what it might mean to him.

Curtis replied, "No, no, absolutely not."

I probed. "What was it like, in the beginning, getting used to health care aides coming into your home?"

"I think even touching on that is a sore point of mine," Curtis replied. "I'm a very private person."

"I remember when Olivia, the home care manager for the program at that time, was surprised that I was only asking for one hour. It was because home care was an intrusion to my life really. It was a great help, but I tell you very honestly, I was not looking forward to the person ringing the doorbell in the morning. I just felt it was intruding into our lives. I sometimes had to do more to help the health care aide who came in. They weren't always competent to do the work. I recall one worker that I had to help with positioning Mary into the bathtub with a hydraulic chair, all with the water pressure moving up and down. They should have been able to do that as that was the point of the hydraulic chair. I could do it on my own. She did bathe, dry, and dress Mary, but I had to be there to help. And that was," he stopped for a moment. "It was enough."

"That was good for that time in our lives. After the second stroke, my privacy was non-existent. We needed more outside help. I decided that I would bring her home from St. John's Center, the rehab place. In there she was in Violet Gardens, in the last room of the corridor, alone. She couldn't push a button, she couldn't ask for help. The only moveable part of her body was her neck, her head. So, she was a prisoner. She was probably worse off than a prisoner so to speak, you know?"

He didn't really want an answer. I slowly nodded as I listened.

"I spent twelve hours there every day for six months, from 8 AM until 8 PM, and I thought to myself, this cannot go on. This is almost like a death sentence and this is when I asked Olivia to have a meeting with me. Olivia was sitting there where you are now, Kim." He gave a slight nod toward me. "I was sitting right here and I described how I, quite a naïve, inexperienced person in the total home care and helping world, saw that it can work. I asked her to honestly tell me if she thought I was crazy thinking that I could take Mary home and look after her as I so desperately wanted. She agreed with me and said, 'You can do it and you will be able to transfer her alone.' At which point I thought *she* was crazy, so I said, 'How will I able to do it alone? Mary's a dead weight.'"

"So she sent me to this medical supply store. I went right away and they were amazingly helpful. I had the lift system installed and when everything was cleared for discharge Mary came home. Now the key to this, that's a very important thing what I'm saying to you now, the key person to the success of this operation from the financial point of view was a lady who worked for the home care program—the case manager. She was the one who would help us get home care arranged. She interviewed me for about two hours. Completely, I mean she got a clear picture of my emotional, my physical, and any other potential problems and she said to me, 'I will recommend that it should be approved.' Now why was she the key? I could have taken Mary from St. John's, you know, signing their necessary document that I had requested a discharge at my own risk. But then I would have to pay for home care from one of the private agencies because if they didn't approve it thinking I took her home against the recommendation of our doctor and the care home, the public system would not approve us. That would have cost me a fortune. So I was very grateful and this is one of the two persons who supported me. And, you know, my age was against me. Back in 2001, I was seventy-four."

"Olivia, the manager of the home care program and essentially my case manager's boss, asked me to prepare a proposal for her, for the home care program that I would list what I could do and what I needed to get Mary care at home instead of where she was—in St. John's. That was a serious business because I had to think very carefully that, now here is my wife whom I knew at that time for fifty-one years. I knew her daily procedures and desires and what not. So I prepared something, I kept it on my computer. I asked for the exact amount of care I thought we needed. I listed the equipment we had like a simple bath seat, raised toilet seat, and grab bars from before Mary went to St. John's. I said I needed a hydraulic chair and a walker. I think that showed them I was serious and I planned this out."

Curtis was a thoughtful and resourceful caregiver for Mary. He was organized and took charge of their situation. He was the hub. He felt supported with his home care and was determined to get what he needed. His diligent advocacy served them well, but not all family caregivers have the same capacity and energy levels for advocacy. Sometimes, that is what makes the difference between getting what you need or not.

I routinely ask family caregivers I come into contact with a question and it is the same one I often ask my research study participants at the end of our interview. I ask them, "Can you give me one suggestion or comment for health decision-makers or policy-makers about ways our home care system could be better for you?" They are quick to share their ideas. There is some variation in their responses but most of them can be grouped around a few key areas. One common request is more support in general for family caregivers—there simply is not enough. A second is more access to accurate and timely information; often family caregivers feel that they are in the dark. A third is more compassion and understanding from health care providers, including nurses and physicians. Family caregivers feel they are poorly understood and given little credence or time for listening. Lastly, they tell me appropriate respite from home care is sorely needed. Support, access to accurate and timely information, compassionate engagement with health care providers, and respect are themes found in most caregiver stories throughout this book. Respite was alluded to, but some stories illustrate the significance of respite as a necessary service for family caregivers more so than others. For this reason, I have included it here as part of the spectrum of home care services.

CHAPTER FIVE

Respite

"I had to do a lot of advocating and that was very difficult. If I needed a break out of town, it was near impossible; it certainly would have been easier for me if home care would have been able or willing to provide more respite in the home. I tried to get him placed in a care home but they didn't want to take him because his care requirements were too great. I had to push for the respite I did receive with everybody—home care, the care home, hospital administrator, and my MLA. And I had to keep following up."

—Myrna

RESPITE CARE, TEMPORARY ASSISTANCE DESIGNED to provide a break for full-time caregivers, rarely meets the needs of family caregivers. I know that's a pretty big statement, but my observations as a nurse, home care nurse, administrator, and researcher bear this out. Often thought of as an add-on, rather than an integral part of a family's care package, respite care seems designed to suit the system, rather than the caregivers themselves.

Part of the problem is that respite is a service designed for the family caregiver, rather than the client to whom all other home and health care services are allocated. While home care is designed to meet an "unmet need" (those needs family or friends cannot provide) of a person requiring care, respite is provided for the family caregiver's rest and relaxation, as a general break from caregiving responsibilities. Sometimes, during respite periods, the person being cared for doesn't need any assistance, which means that the respite worker just needs to be present to ensure that the client is safe. Unfortunately, the mechanisms to fund this type of care aren't always in place.

Respite Care: What Is It?

There are two main types of respite: in-home respite and out-of-home respite. In-home respite is provided to a client and family when the family member already has home care. It is designed to give the caregiver a short break to rest, run errands, or take part in leisure or social activities. There are, however, instances when no other home care services are provided other than respite, which is often the only chance a family caregiver has to get out of the house. This is particularly true if a loved one cannot be left alone for any period of time.

With out-of-home respite, the family member receiving care and support is placed in another program or facility to give the caregiver a break. While a client may be out of home for other services such as a day program, rehabilitation, or other therapeutic service, that is not considered respite for the caregiver, but rather necessary services for the care recipient. Out-of-home respite can be offered on a short-term, recurring basis or in the longer term, ranging from a few weeks to a month. Long-term, out-of-home respite might take place on a recurring basis—one a month, say, or every few months—but mostly it occurs on an as-needed basis.

Finding the right support for in-home respite depends on the availability and education of certain types of workers. That's what makes it so challenging. There's no specific education for respite care workers, which means that this type of care is often provided by aides—people who are educated to handle personal care, give medications, and provide some treatments under the direction of a nurse, for example. If the client has mobility or toileting needs, then a health care aide is required. If they require a higher skill level, then a nurse should be deployed. Often, however, health care aides and nurses tend to be over-qualified for most respite shifts where no personal care, hands-on assistance, or medical treatments are needed, which is a poor use of health care resources if indeed a health care aide or a nurse even had availability in their schedule.

The home care program administration is not often keen to use health care aides or nurses for a "just in case scenario" as they are more appropriately used for clients who need their skill level for hands-on care and treatments. For many respite shifts, a lesser skilled person is appropriate as the need is for someone to be present for safety, cueing, or companionship so the client is not left unattended. This is not an unreasonable approach from the health care system's perspective; however, it is problematic for clients and family caregivers when they can't access respite workers.

The titles and roles of support workers and assistant-level workers in home and community care can be confusing to families. "Health care aides," "personal care attendants," and "personal care assistants" are terms that often mean the same thing: a non-regulated care provider with eight to sixteen weeks of training in personal care. Non-regulated means not subject to a regulatory body as nurses, physicians, physical and occupational therapists, and pharmacists are. A non-regulated worker's role and scope varies between jurisdictions. Typically, they follow a plan of care developed by a regulated professional, such as a case manager or a nurse. These non-regulated workers do not make clinical judgments that would change the course of treatment or plan of care without consulting a supervisor, typically a regulated professional.

The terms "support worker" and "companion worker" are also used, as are titles such as "home support worker," "respite worker," or "companion sitter." Support workers and companions typically don't provide hands-on care, but they may do light housekeeping, meal prep (but not feeding), as well as provide companionship and facilitate leisure activities. It is important that clients and their family caregivers know the difference between the available staff members so they can not only understand the limits and scope of what each can do but also so they are able to advocate effectively for what they need in terms of respite support for their loved one.

Myrna

By the time respite was instituted Dad could do little for himself, either independently or with assistance. Mom had no concerns about her in-home respite hours. Dad's needs were extensive and it was clear that he required a health care aide at a minimum. So, every Tuesday and Friday from 10:00 AM until noon, home care provided respite care at the personal care aide level. Even now, seventeen years after his death, I can recall the timing of Dad's respite care. I remember the urgency we felt every Tuesday and Friday as we rushed to get out of the house as soon as the caregiver arrived. Most mornings we had to leave right away so we had time to do all of the errands—shop for groceries, get gas, attend appointments, or do whatever was on Mom's agenda—and make it home by noon when the caregiver's shift ended.

It was out-of-home respite that caused Mom's excessive stress. Once a year, she would take a trip, either to visit me and my family in Alberta or to my sister and her family in the United States. Mom's only break, this annual excursion was necessary for her own rest and recovery. Not only did she have to get the placement for respite pre-arranged, she had to update Dad's care plan book—a book we kept at home with all of Dad's routines, notes on particular challenges like how to feed him without choking him, what his facial expressions meant, and the importance of giving him liquids to avoid a urinary tract infection. These things seem basic, but without Mom noting all of Dad's care requirements and how to care for him effectively, things would fall apart. She had to ensure they knew he needed puréed food and she would pre-prepare snacks to leave for him. Sometimes when they wanted to place Dad in a facility far from our hometown, Mom had to fight to convince the administration as to why it was not possible. With a lack of staffing at meals and night-time, Mom also hired private nurses she knew who could care for Dad by providing his supper feeding and care overnight.

I got the chance to interview Mom when we were on a family winter vacation some years after Dad had passed. I wanted time alone with her so I could capture her nuanced perspective, rather than rely on my memory. I also didn't want the others chiming in. We were all involved in Dad's life and care in intimate and extensive ways, and we all had our stories. I wanted Mom's version. I wanted to get the full picture of her struggle with out-of-home respite.

We took our coffees out to the patio overlooking the beautiful Caribbean Sea. It was early in the morning before the others were up and we started by recalling some of Dad's personal care workers. We remembered Sheryl—a beautiful singer who sang one of Mom and Dad's favorite songs at his funeral, *There Goes My Everything*. Monica used to come early to have the obligatory coffee with Mom. She was a skilled crocheter who made Mom an exquisite table-cloth. Betty always had lots of stories and knew several of Dad's old friends, so would reminisce with him. He always looked forward to her shifts.

"I was glad to get the care I got," Mom said, "but it was the out-of-home respite that was so hard on me. Trying to go away for a few weeks so I could have a break was very difficult."

"You seemed to have to figure it all out on your own, too. I remember that. No one provided you with information without a lot of digging on your part. Even to prove you were eligible for it."

"Exactly. I had to go to Dr. Hickey, our MLA at the time; I wrote to Maritime Medical [the insurance carrier]; I even went down to Halifax to meet with them. I had to do a lot of advocating at the time and that was very difficult."

"And home care wouldn't provide you any additional care for two weeks?"

"No, no, they wouldn't give us any more care than the two hours he got each day or the four respite hours we could use each week. Not at all." She shook her head and sighed.

Unfortunately, this is not uncommon. In-home respite care is under-resourced and is often provided in small allotments each week—one or two shifts of three to four hours each. I have rarely heard of families getting more than that. There needs to be a combination of both in-home and out-of-home respite and it needs to be much more individualized depending on how heavy the burden of care is on the caregiver. In my mother's case, she was giving Dad at least twelve hours of direct hands-on care every day over and above what the health care aides were providing. She was doing personal care, feeding, treatments, getting Dad drinks, lifting him, and changing his position—it was heavy care for anyone. Getting necessary respite should not be so difficult for family caregivers. Accessing appropriate respite is such a chore that many simply give up and stop asking.

"Do you think it would have been easier for you if home care would have been able or willing to provide respite in the home?"

"Oh, yes for sure. If you could get away for a few weeks to get a break. Yes, absolutely. I had to try and get him placed. It was that or pay for twenty-four hours of care on my own. It just wasn't feasible at the time. I had to push for the respite and keep following up. And near the end, the last few years before Dad died, the nursing homes just weren't equipped to look after someone with his needs. They told me that themselves. They did not offer any other solutions. It was me left problem solving what we were going to do about it."

I remember the family discussing whether or not Mom should go away at all. She didn't want to, but she was exhausted and we— my sisters and I in particular—pushed her to take a break. It was a challenging time. We were worried about Mom and we were worried about Dad. We girls knew it was important for her to get away because we could see when she was getting exhausted. She would talk about how tired she was and that she just couldn't be bothered fighting. She would sound depressed and resigned. Then afterward, she would feel refreshed, and we could see that, too. So as much as we knew how challenging it was for Mom to arrange respite, she needed it. Because my brother and his wife were the only siblings close by and were back and forth several times a week seeing to household things Mom and Dad needed, they got a little break as well.

"Towards the end of Dad's life, in the last year of my caregiving— and it was the last time I went away," Mom said, "I wanted him in the hospital. It was the only place I felt was suitable for him. But they wouldn't take him."

I was thinking about that, too: how ridiculous it was that we could not seem to get two weeks for Mom to have a break. Our family was not all that different from others I knew in caregiving situations all across the country. Being part of national home care not-for-profit boards, I heard similar stories from other home care leaders at our meetings, as well as from caregivers in Alberta, where I was Director of our home care organization. People could not access enough respite, if they did not need hands-on care from a health care aide or nurse, lesser skilled companions would be sent—but they didn't always have skills—language, similar hobbies, knowledge of favorite card games—that satisfied family caregivers. Out-of-home respite beds were few and the waiting lists were long. Respite care is not as valued as it needs to be. It is a necessary service just like hands-on care or rehabilitation.

"The placement coordinator, the nurse in that role, insisted he go into a long-term care home, rather than the hospital. I was willing to hire our own private duty registered nurse who knew Dad and have her be there for night shifts, when there was less staff and Nanna would be with him every afternoon, but they wouldn't even permit me to do that, so we had no options."

This, even though the nursing homes were saying that Dad's needs were too extensive and that they didn't have the staff to budget to the hours of care Dad would need each day. This is the essence of this paradox. Family caregivers toil, they learn how to care for their loved ones and keep them at home with a little support from home care. The condition of the client deteriorates, their needs grow, and when they need respite placement for a short break their requirements have gone beyond what the system will provide. This is reality. It is asinine.

Mom shook her head, recalling the struggle. "I knew it wasn't good, but that was all they would allow—care in the long-term care home that knew they couldn't properly care for him. It was ridiculous."

I nodded. This was small-town Nova Scotia; Mom and Dad had been part of the community forever. She had been a nurse at the hospital for a long time, so she knew many of the nurses she was dealing with, either first-hand or through me and my sister (we were, after all, a family of nurses). Given the connections we had—certainly more than most—it was mind-boggling that we were out of our depth. I was entrenched in this system out west, and active in high-level policy circles at both the government and health system levels. I was even a board member for a national community care organization. And I could do little to help my own family navigate these barriers.

Situations like this are a particularly stressful part of the caregiving process. Powerless against systems and bureaucracy, family caregivers feel defeated. They find it hard to take any kind of action because all of their efforts are for naught, and that leads them to a place of "Why bother?" That's a natural response from caregivers who are already exhausted—physically, mentally, and emotionally—and feeling alone in their journey. Yet, they need to muster the strength to keep going and provide the care and support to their loved one every day. That does not change, despite any new arising challenges.

Thinking of Mom and Dad's situation, no one seemed able to reach through the barriers. The mechanisms just weren't in place for appropriate respite. I recall how stressful it was. Mom was willing to put in place extra nurses at her own cost and the fact that they would not allow that—without a good explanation—nor offer any other solutions was not only stressful but maddening. People—other family, friends, and even home care nurses and case managers, the very people who should be supporting family caregivers—have little insight into the stress of family caregivers. When they need some relief from caregiving, most are at their breaking point. It is frustrating that there is a failure to see this. Another difficult thing was that we knew long-term care was not equipped to handle someone with Dad's high needs, but also there were no options other than the acute care hospital—not a reasonable solution from the health system's perspective. This scenario plays out across Canada. Sad to say it's much the same nearly two decades later.

Still, at our lovely breakfast overlooking the ocean, Mom took a sip of her coffee and continued, "I couldn't get him in palliative care either, he wasn't appropriate for that. They had no idea where to place him and they didn't seem too interested in helping me find a solution. They also didn't seem to understand how these breaks were so important to caregivers. They just didn't get it."

Mom paused and shook her head before continuing, "Some awful things were said to me. I'll never forget it. Like the time I wanted him placed in the hospital, he was too high needs by then for long-term care. The placement coordinator said they were going to place him in a spot that opened 100 miles away from home—in Pugwash! She was a nurse and she said, 'Well, what do you care, Myrna? You're not going to be here anyway'—those were exactly her words!"

"Well, I just said to her right away, 'Of course I care! He has family who want to see him, a mother who needs to be able to see him.' Nanna was about eighty-seven at the time and she would go and sit with him every afternoon for three or four hours, remember that?"

I shifted in my chair to get out of the sun. "Yes, I do remember. I was so disgusted at that nurse. How can anyone say something like that, let alone think it? And these are the people who are supposed to help ease your burden."

"Exactly."

"When you think back, is there anything you have ever thought about that would have made a difference, or lightened your load?"

"Easier respite. If a person could get a break easier, maybe two or three times a year. But I only ever was able to get two weeks a year. Even that it was difficult to get it. Proper respite would have made a *big* difference." Mom drew out her annunciation to stress just how big. "Yes, that would have made a big difference."

Caregivers regularly say they don't mind doing what they are doing. They accept it. But when they can't get a break, and when respite is not there for them, it is hard. It pisses them off. It makes it hard to continue the day in and day out relentlessness of caregiving if they can't look forward to even a short break.

It's not there for people who need it most. I think it is only going to get worse for families as we try to keep everyone in the community and have family pick up so much of the slack. Home care does a little, but only a few hours in a day. So much falls on the spouse and the rest of the family.

At this point, the system cannot take care of the sickest people who are well looked after at home by the family caregiver with support from home care. There is definitely something wrong with this picture.

I turned to my mother. "There was no respite towards the end for you. If Dad hadn't died when he did, I don't think you ever would have gotten him in anywhere for respite."

Mom agreed.

We both knew they couldn't look after him properly in long-term care. And they (the care home, or the health authority) weren't willing to put the resources in, either, so they *could* look after someone like Dad. Our physician tried to advocate to get Dad into the hospital, as well. She also knew that the care home wouldn't be able to cope. Neither Mom nor she could get through to anyone. No one would do anything for them or even try to think outside of the box—citing rules and regulations and all of that. There was no will to even attempt to try and fix what was not working and it is still that way. But it's not their family. The lack of respite is often the hardest thing for Mom, and caregivers like her, to deal with.

Respite is not there for people who need it most. If a person's care is too advanced for long-term care, there is no other option. It seems counter-intuitive that we are able to look after people at home with exceptionally high needs, yet the care homes and even the hospitals can't properly look after them. It is a problem that is progressing to even worse states as families take on even greater care needs at home.

Respite seems to be there when the person is not that badly off or their needs are not too high, but it's not there for people who need it most: the ones who are really critical or have advanced levels of need. Administrators think hospitals shouldn't have to provide it and long-term care is so structured around a few hours of care a day that their funding levels can't meet the need. The Covid-19 pandemic of 2020 has certainly shone a light on the magnitude of care issues for people needing both long-term care and home care.

At this point, we have a system that cannot take care of the sickest people, many of whom are well looked after at home by the family caregiver with support from home care. There are problems with so many aspects of care, from structural and process issues to policy problems and societal ignorance. The issue is underpinned by a funding issue with no apparent political will to address it.

Then Mom suddenly thought about the book we called Dad's Care Book. It had everything in it. His routine, what he could do, the kind of assistance he needed, cues for him, how to feed him. What he liked and didn't like.

The last thing Mom said before I turned off the tape and we went to the beach was, "I should have kept Dad's Care Book after he died. It was always updated with everything. I don't know why we ever got rid of it."

As I got out of my chair, I mumbled, "I don't know." But I do know. Seventeen years later, I knew why we didn't. It was too raw immediately afterward. We couldn't see then why we would ever want to look at it and remember such strain and sadness, and what was not how Mom and Dad wanted to live. None of us had envisioned our life like that. Why would we want to relive it after he was gone? That's why we didn't save it.

CHAPTER SIX

Information Needs

"I love you enough to research your condition and your medications and to pester the doctors and pharmacists for answers. Because I love you, I continue to seek answers that will improve your quality of life."

—Penny

In Search of Comprehensive, Consistent Care

"IF I ONLY KNEW YOU when I was caring for," people will say, before going on to tell me how they felt at a loss about where to turn for help. Not surprising. Finding accurate and timely information on services, resources, and equipment to make their lives a little easier is one of the biggest challenges caregivers face.

I've met people who struggled with loved ones at home—some whose family members died at home—with virtually no home care or community support. Not because they didn't need it, but because no one ever told them about it. This can happen even in cases where families are already connected to the health care system. Either no one told them anything about home care or other community supports, or the information received was inaccurate, incomplete, or discouraging. When family caregivers hear statements like "Don't bother calling home care as services are so limited you won't qualify" or "They're so stretched you will be waiting for a long time to get anything," they believe them. After all, they have no reason to question these well-meaning, but ill-informed, health care professionals.

All too often, by the time family caregivers interact with the health system, their loved one's condition has advanced to the point where they can no longer cope. They need additional support. Not only hands-on physical care for their loved one, but information such as where to find equipment or medical supplies like adult diapers, as well as places where funding for these items might be available. What they find is a system that is fragmented and siloed. Fragmented in that there is usually lack of collaboration between departments and agencies. And siloed, indicating a system where people work within closed environments—often completely unaware or ignorant of other parts that are equally closed off, making communication and coordination virtually impossible.

Health professionals who work in hospitals with more acute care rarely have an understanding of or interest in what goes on after the patient leaves. They are busy, in tune with their own setting, and naïve as to what happens in other sectors. However, this can lead to distress for caregivers who don't know what they don't know. They reasonably assume that their trusted health professional will provide them with the information they need.

Family caregivers have a right to expect a system that offers comprehensive consistent care, rather than the current approach that often leaves them dependent on their own resourcefulness. Health care professionals should be concerned with more than just meeting the immediate needs of their clients. That is, they should approach the situation from a holistic perspective, one that considers the impact of the illness on both the client and their family caregiver who will likely be providing care well into the future. This holistic approach would also include access to community supports and services that will help them manage well—usually at home.

Family caregivers need to be given accurate information on available resources and services at their first contact with the health care system, whether it is with a family physician or home care case manager. Often on the first visit the needs of the client are identified. It is usually clear that the family caregiver is going to be providing care and support to their loved one at home. The right information would better equip them to make decisions about the care and other supports they will need.

One problem is that sometimes the caregiver doesn't recognize their role and they may not appreciate the extent of the care and support they will be providing. It may not be until they are well into their caregiving role that their information needs become obvious. The family physician is usually one of the first points, or only point, of contact. It behooves physicians to be proactive with the family caregiver. Even a preliminary information sheet of resources for the caregiver to access would be helpful. Phone numbers for places like equipment providers, the home care program, and the local agency serving family caregivers would be extremely helpful. Most states and provinces have agencies that focus on the needs of family caregiving and there are national organizations as well. These organizations usually offer everything from information sessions to education and courses on family caregiving, as well as peer support. They are generally well connected to other caregiving supports within a community and can offer referrals.

Finding Support in Your Community

Most families don't want a swinging door of service providers, which can seem like an invasion of their space and privacy. However, the right services at the right time can be a life saver. You will need accurate and current information to help you make the best choices.

Here are some first steps:

In-person

Access a transition worker at your local health unit. **Case managers, social workers, or community resource specialists** can help you find the right resources in your own community. The individuals who can help you are called different things in different agencies so ask who is available to help you find resources to help you care for your loved one.

Then ask questions like:

Do you have any print information on various programs I can take with me?

What does each program offer? How do I access it? What is the phone number? Who is the best person to talk to?

If you or your loved one are an older person, ask about local organizations that provide programs and services for older people. Ask friends who work in health care where you can find information. Don't be shy. Ask your physician or a nurse in the doctor's office and hospital. If they don't know, then push them to look into it for you while you wait. Look up "Home Care" or "Community Care."

Once you connect with a good resource, you will likely find it easier to get referred to others for information and support.

Home care

Home care programs provide care workers. **Personal care assistants or health care aides**—they are called by different titles in different jurisdictions—have a short education (usually 306 months) and are unregulated. **Nurses** may also be provided; they are regulated professionals. Different home care programs provide different levels of service. Who provides your care depends on what you need, based on a thorough assessment that usually takes sixty to ninety minutes.

The **assessment** may be carried out by a regulated health care professional, usually a nurse but possibly a social worker or a rehabilitation professional. They may be called a **Case Manager**. Think about where you need help to care for your loved one and ask for the support you need.

Some questions to ask are:

What kinds of care providers are available? Is there a cost? What kinds of things can I get help with?

Ask about things like personal care such as bathing, dressing, toileting. What about meal preparation or feeding? Or laundry?

Can I break up the amount of time I am eligible for? What makes us eligible for home care? Can I get care at night-time? What about respite so I can leave the home without worrying? How many times a week can I get that?

Are private services available? If I want more than is provided by the government home care program, can I "top up" by purchasing private care? What private home care companies are in the area? Do you have any information on them? Do they also work with home care?

(Continued)

Note on home care: In many jurisdictions, home care is contracted by the public (government) home care program to private service provider agencies who employ health care aides and personal care attendants and in some cases the nurses. What the public program contracts out varies by jurisdiction. The private service providers under government contract have to prove they meet specific standards. This is usually done by various reporting and auditing regulations by the contracting government agency.

Online information

Accessibility to information for caregivers has improved with the internet, but the quality of the material you unearth will depend on your ability to search well, so being somewhat internet savvy and having a little bit of knowledge about what to look for can help.

A single, comprehensive, and regularly updated website targeted to family caregivers would be a fantastic resource, but information is often found in different places. However, there are organizations that exist solely to support caregivers, and they usually have good websites. As well, most programs and services will have a website, and many link to other community supports and online resources.

Search terms you might try:

Family caregiving in [my neighborhood or city]
Supports for
Resources for
Home care program
Supports for seniors
Home care
Meal program

Meal delivery
Services for care at home
Private home care
Home support services
Home health care equipment
Home care supplies

The terms home health, home care, home support might all yield different results but are terms that are sometimes used interchangeably.

Be aware of the publisher of the site you are looking at. Is it the organization's own site or a third-party site promoting something? Is it a government site? A good tip is that the organization's name or government identifier will actually appear in their website's name.

Activity:
Regardless of where you are on your caregiving journey, begin a "Resource File."

Be organized: create a system that works as you may hear about supports that you don't need now but may be helpful down the road. Having a file will at least offer a starting point.

Gathering Information

The same preliminary information that your physicians ought to provide you could also be provided by any health professional who is in a position to see family caregivers, including home care case managers. This information should be shared on the first visit. When a client starts on home care, the case manager, usually a registered nurse, does an intake assessment. She gathers information on the client's health status and functional ability. Can the client walk and feed himself? How does she manage in the bathroom? What level and type of assistance is required?

The family caregiver should be present for this assessment and sometimes will be asked about their willingness and ability to care for their loved one. They may be asked questions about what they do for the person now, and if they have any support system in place. The caregiver is often early on in their caregiving role and so may be coping well at this stage. However, beyond the initial assessment there is rarely any intentional follow up with the caregiver. The care the client requires is the focus of home care. A brochure or information sheet with details on what caregiving is, what the caregiver can expect, and useful community resources that are focused on caregivers would be helpful. Then, when a caregiver is feeling stressed or needing particular information, they would at least have a starting point.

Health professionals rarely consider the specific needs of the caregiver since their primary focus is the client with health problems. Preliminary information would let the caregiver know there are supports available and how to access them. They would be in a better position to take charge of their situation and ask questions proactively. The health professional may not have immediate answers but most would be inclined to seek out resources if the caregiver expresses a need.

The Starting Point

Questions to ask your health care provider or physician:
- Where can I find equipment like wheelchairs or walkers?
- Where do I look for help in the home, like home care?
- Is there any support for me, like an organization for family caregivers?
- Where would I look for funding programs that might be available to help pay for equipment or supplies?

What to Expect from Home Care

Caregivers often don't know what to expect from home care. What services are available? What can they negotiate? It's frustrating for caregivers to receive so little information, particularly when such information is available but not well advertised. When I was doing my research with family caregivers, I provided many of them with basic information they already should have been informed about, such as where they could access additional equipment (special beds, chairs, cushions, or mechanical lifts) and what programs were available to assist with either costs or equipment rental. They might not have been told about such things if it had been some time since their case manager visited the home, or if their case manager was unaware of escalating needs (some of which could have been avoided if the family caregiver was receiving proper support to begin with). I found that family caregivers respond with a range of different emotions when they finally get information that can help them. They may feel relief, anger, or defeat. Relief that they now have *some* information, anger if the information comes too late, or defeat because they are so weary from their constant struggle for support.

All decisions should be shared between the client, family caregiver, and home care, but if a family member doesn't understand that they might be able to refuse some services, like a bath assist, or ask for something different, like respite, it may not be offered. Clients sometimes go months or years without fully understanding how home care works for them. They're marginalized because they can't ask for something they don't know exists. At the same time, they may be getting services they don't feel they need, which essentially is a mismanagement of resources perhaps causing some clients to go without. It saddens me to see what the lack of information does to families, how quickly they feel defeated when they cannot get the information they need, and how it isolates them from receiving adequate support.

Donelle didn't know she could have had a licensed practical nurse doing night-time care. The home care case manager instead offered her a health care aide, not recognizing that Donelle would still have to get up at midnight and four in the morning to give her husband his IV medications—tasks that are beyond the skill set of health care aides but that LPNs can do on their own under a physician's order. Donelle kindly refused the health care aide for the night shift as she felt it wouldn't meet their needs. Donelle, being a health care professional, had the wherewithal to problem solve the night shifts herself. She called upon friends who were nurses or pharmacists to stay a few nights a week with her husband so she could sleep and they could provide all the care that was required, including giving him his medications. The other nights she managed on her own.

She was exhausted. Then she discovered she actually could have asked to have LPNs at night to administer her husband's medication. She stumbled on this news quite by accident, with a different case manager who presented more comprehensive information. If Donelle hadn't received this information, she would have continued to improvise a situation that could have led to several negative outcomes. Apart from the discomfort of having to rely on friends for such a long period of time, Donelle could have become completely exhausted to a point where she could have been unable to continue caring for her husband. Perhaps in her exhausted state she might even have made an error with his medication. "If they only told me all of what I could choose from I could have made better decisions," she said. "I didn't want more than they could give, I only wanted what we should have had in the first place."

Home Care Equipment

When information about home care equipment is lacking, caregivers are at higher risk for personal injury, especially back and joint injuries. When a bed is too low to assist someone with bathing, positioning, or moving about, the caregiver will likely develop back strain. Beds and chairs often need to be replaced, adjusted, or modified to make caregiving safer. While it may be somewhat costly, neglecting these adjustments may turn out to be a case of penny-wise, pound-foolish. Failure to invest in what is needed to make caregiving as safe as possible can result in injuries that, in turn, can create additional challenges that may affect the caregiver's ability to provide care. Basic information about the availability of assistive devices for the bedroom or bathroom, mechanical lifts, and other items needs to be provided early so caregivers have an opportunity to consider what would be most helpful in terms of costs and practical implications.

Many creative adjustments can be carried out to make caregiving easier and safer for the caregiver. For example, installing a pole into the floor can allow the person being cared for to help themselves with moving and standing. A towel bar or grab bar securely attached to the wall parallel to the bed can be used as an anchor for a belt or strap, a handy way to assist with movement, including pulling oneself to sitting. A stool or seat in the shower is a safety measure that can mean the difference between having a shower or a bed-bath. A towel bar by the bathroom sink provides support while using the sink. Even plates and bowls with suction rings on the bottom can make eating easier and a little more dignified as it is easier to get food onto spoons or forks without the dishes slipping. There are also adult bibs, clothing and shoes with Velcro closures, and cushions for seating that all make caregiving a little more manageable.

Of course, there may be aesthetic and practical implications, such as space and how public a room is in the home. As well, these devices need to be properly installed to withstand the weight that will be applied. Nevertheless, with a little bit of ingenuity, adjustments can be safely made to help both the caregiver and the individual being cared for.

Specialized medical equipment can be very expensive and is often not fully covered by government or third-party insurance programs. Larger equipment such as hospital-style beds or mechanical devices to help lift and move loved ones require adequate space. When families are using home care or other health care services, they are not always made aware of some equipment options. Unfortunately, it is sometimes left up to the family caregiver to ask what might be available; this is another instance where it is hard to know what to ask for if you don't know what might be possible. Starting with a question like, "Are there any home care equipment suppliers in this area? Are there any equipment loan programs?" is often enough to open up the conversation and get some information. If not, looking to the internet and local telephone directory is a good place to start. Once caregivers get connected—even to one resource—this can lead to other referrals that often snowball in a good way for the caregiver.

If home care staff are assigned to provide care in the home, the case manager will do a health risk and safety assessment to ensure the environment is safe for care providers—particularly because occupational health and safety laws legislate policies to protect employees. (Family members aren't considered employees, so there are no similar laws protecting them.) Any equipment the home care staff will use will also be assessed for safety.

Jeanette

I recently had a conversation with Jeanette at a caregiver appreciation and self-care event. A participant in one of my workshops, she updated me on how things were going caring for her husband, who had Alzheimer's disease. Unfortunately, Jeanette's spouse was deteriorating quite rapidly—both his incontinence and his dementia were increasing, although he still had the occasional good day.

Home care came for thirty minutes every morning to help him take his medication and get bathed and dressed. Often, he refused to bathe. He wetted or soiled himself so frequently he wore adult diapers. It was a challenge for her to keep him dry and keep up with the laundry. Incontinence products are very expensive, although some people may have coverage through extended health insurance plans or local jurisdictions to help obtain supplies at a cheaper or no cost if they qualify. Jeanette's husband qualified—although it was a long time into his incontinence before she discovered and accessed the program.

"He wears the Attends and I get them from the health authority," Jeanette told me.

"Through AADL?" I asked her. AADL is the Alberta Aids to Daily Living program that provides funding for basic medical equipment and disposable supplies, including adult diapers. Need is based on assessment and it's a helpful program for clients with long-term and chronic health conditions.

"Yes, I think that's the program. They give me his diapers and boosters. But they won't give me enough boosters. It is ridiculous. I don't want too many diapers but they keep giving me boxes of these things."

Her purse hung off her shoulder. She was holding a small plate of appetizers and balancing a juice glass while making gestures with her other hand as she spoke. She said even telling me her story caused her to relive her frustration.

"Do you know why I can't get any more boosters? I don't understand it. It would save them money. That's all I need is more boosters. I don't want more diapers. I can't get them to understand."

I assumed she meant separate pads that were placed inside the diaper or pull-up brief, but I wanted to be sure. "I am sorry. What are boosters? I am not familiar with that term."

"They are like big pads that go in the diaper." She puts her plate and purse down so she can gesture with two hands. She holds her hands about a foot apart and makes a motion that looks like a tube. "They are this big and you just put them in the diaper. They absorb the pee and I just need to change that, not the whole diaper."

"Oh, I understand now. I didn't know they were called that."

"It is easier for me to replace the booster than change the whole diaper and he needs the boosters. With just the diaper he gets so wet, his clothes get saturated and his skin breaks down from the pee. This is way better and cheaper."

"I am so frustrated. I never have enough of the boosters. They tell me I can't have more boosters because there's a limit—a quota for the things. But there is on the diapers, too, and I don't use all that they give me. I talked to other people and they tell me they have the same problem. Then I hear when people die, they have to look for places who will take boxes of diapers because they have so many left over."

I could see that she was feeling defeated that no one was hearing her at AADL. I nodded as she spoke. When she finally obtained some help, she wasn't able to get enough of the right product (pads, more absorbent and less expensive than the full pull up), yet she was being sent an over-supply of the more expensive full pull up men's brief that she didn't use. Frustratingly for Jeanette, the rules under the current system did not allow her to return or exchange the pull ups for pads. It was much easier for her and her husband to exchange a wet pad for a dry one and reuse the pull up. Her solution was less expensive and easier on her health. Yet, it didn't seem to be an option.

"I keep calling them but they don't seem to get it."

"So, you call the office and just talk to who answers the phone?"

"Yeah. It's the people I always talk to."

"I wonder if you could ask to speak to the authorizer? That's the health professional who came out and did your assessment and who approved what you were eligible for. If you talk directly to that person you can likely ask for another assessment. Tell them that what they give you helps to a degree, but your husband's health is changing and you need to be reassessed to see if there are other things that could help you."

I gave her some words to use that could prompt action:

- "What we have is not working for us."
- "My husband needs to be reassessed as I can't continue with what we are doing."
- "I need someone to come out and see what is going on."

I suggested she call her home care case manager directly and ask for a home visit with the purpose of reassessing the incontinence.

Use the Right Language

Knowing what language to use can help you get prompt action. Here are some other suggestions:
- I am finding that the allotted time is not working for us.
- I am not able to [INSERT the specific tasks here, e.g. "lift"] him anymore.
- I am physically and mentally exhausted and need a break.
- I need more care for the [SPECIFIC TIME, e.g. "evening"].
- I would like to change the time of day the caregiver comes.

Be as specific as you can.

Caregivers can be uncomfortable advocating strongly for what they need because many fear they will lose what care they have if they are asking for too much or burdening the system. This is not the case. However, it is a reality I have witnessed time and again. If a caregiver uses language that the system uses, people will take action because they more easily understand what the caregiver is asking for.

The action might be an answer to a question or providing information or help to obtain outside resources or equipment. If the caregiver doesn't ask or is not specific about what could make a difference, the case manager may not be aware of their problems.

Each case manager's knowledge about, and their connection to, community resources varies. The variation might be related to their experience in home care, their education, or their level of compassion for their clients and passion for their work. If a case manager doesn't know the answer to a caregiver's question or where to find particular services, equipment, or supplies, they should be proactive and investigate. It is part of their role. If they don't, then clients and family caregivers miss out on what's available to them. It is a problem that leads to inequitable services for clients and leaves family caregivers more than a little frustrated. There are also situations where no one has taken the time to make sure information on services, resources, or caregiver support is organized for the user and that it gets into their hands. Not only are these scenarios problematic, but they may be unethical, if not immoral. Unethical as inequities can put family caregivers at risk because they're either not getting enough support or they are not getting the right support. Immoral, because it is not right that a caregiver suffers increased burden, exhaustion, or even injury due to inaction or inattention.

Jeanette was frustrated, weary to the point of giving up. How could the people administering the program not see how preposterous this all was?

Faulty Assumptions in Caregiving

Family caregivers would be more empowered and enabled to cope better if they were equipped with knowledge. Sometimes, information is available in a format that's not accessible to some family caregivers, such as online only. Not everyone is technologically connected or web-savvy.

Information might also be inaccessible because of assumptions made by health care professionals and decision-makers. For example, some home care leaders believe if they inform people of all of the services they provide, they'll be inundated with requests. This sort of attitude is all too prevalent. I've heard home care leaders and case managers alike say things like, "If clients know all that we *could* do, they would ask for it all and we can't do that. We don't have the resources to give everything to everyone." In my experience, that is not the case; most clients and family members want only what they need. To assume otherwise is a cynical view of human nature and can prohibit comprehensive care. Most caregivers are reasonable people who want the best care for their loved one, and things that will make their life easier. Access to the supports and services that are available to them can make the difference between coping and crashing. Most would rather not be reliant on all of the services and equipment that are necessary to care for their loved one and keep them as safe and comfortable at home for as long as possible. Their new normal is not normal at all.

In the days when I was Director of We Care Home Health Services in Edmonton, a service provider organization under contract to the local government home care program, many discussions about supports and services occurred at monthly meetings with all of the service provider organizations and the local government home care leadership. We talked about, among other things, what kind of printed material to leave in a client's home, such as instructions for health care aides or nurses and client care plans—basically forms documenting the services that were approved for each client. Some decision-makers, home care administrators, and even case managers believed it would be easier if we provided a standard, itemized list that could be checked off as services were authorized by the case manager. Others believed if this were the case, clients and families would feel obliged to have whatever was on the list regardless of need, even though home care is individualized.

Most caregivers I talk with only want what is really needed. They are often overwhelmed with too many people coming to their homes already, as home care feels not only like an invasion of privacy but also one more thing they need to work around.

Penny

Penny told me about a conversation she had when she was trying to obtain a particular piece of equipment from home care.

"We had no help 'til Demetri had been in bed for about a year and a half. Then, at one point, I had wanted a lift for him, so he could pull himself up, you know?" She mimicked the movement with her arm.

"The trapeze?"

"Yes, exactly. And the case manager said, 'Oh, well, we don't give those unless we're also giving a hospital bed.' I went on to tell her, 'Well maybe we should go that route. Maybe we should go to the hospital bed.' The case manager gasped and said 'Oh! Oh, no! Oh no! He's gotta be in bed at least 80% of the time!' And I said, 'He is!'"

I remember the look on Penny's face—incredulous is the best way to describe it—as she told me how flabbergasted the case worker was. "She continued, shocked, 'But, but if I'm putting in for that, it would look like I'm approving it.' And I said, *so?*"

Penny knew she was getting the run-around. "This is the problem," Penny continued. "It's very difficult to find out what resources really are available. I didn't know what to ask for. I just didn't know. Finally last summer I realized that Demetri's needs had outstripped my skills. I had to have help. And I realized the time had come for him to go into continuing care. So, I spent a few days really sad. I don't like to be not under the same roof as my husband. You know? But I also knew that it would be better for him."

Penny was in a terrible position. When she broached the subject with her husband he seemed relieved, even though he didn't say much. But when he was assessed by the continuing care placement team and asked what he wanted, he said he didn't want placement. Penny was stunned by his answer, but pleased that they were on the same page. They both agreed she needed help.

After a flurry of people finally understanding the couple's situation, they were provided with better services and assigned a case manager who had knowledge of other resources, so they could put different things in place to help them.

"I have an absolutely fantastic team now," Penny told me. "My social worker is Lisa from home care. She's gone out of her way on a number of occasions to help me. The occupational therapist is Joan. Also, very, very good. And you know, they let me know of other resources that are available. So, it made a huge difference. We got the hospital bed in November, I think it was. Of course, home care is not without its problems, but it is better now in a lot of ways."

Penny's experience pushed her to the end of her rope. She believed that placement in continuing care was her only option. Lack of information, and indeed misinformation, meant she wasn't aware of the in-home help available to her. Because the couple wasn't informed about the various care options for which they could be considered, Demetri nearly landed in a long-term care facility prematurely.

This is an instance where services or supports were not offered either because their first case manager was a novice or because she was not proactive enough to find things out on her client's behalf.

Access to the right information should not depend on the resourcefulness, knowledge, and network of an individual case manager. Nor should it depend on the caregiver's own resourcefulness. Caregivers need to be provided with a full range of available programs and services in a comprehensive and cogent manner. What's more, case managers need to be well versed in the available options.

Caregivers without any knowledge of what a home care program might offer can find themselves barely coping. They may be able to cobble together support from family and friends, but solutions are usually day to day or week to week. Without knowledge of the full range of resources, caregivers are rarely able to make the best decisions for their loved ones—or themselves. This may lead them to believe there is no option other than to have their loved one go into continuing care or to the hospital, especially if the person they are caring for is close to dying.

I have talked with too many people who had no idea about the kinds of home care supports they could have accessed. Many caregivers who had these stories usually did not even know that home care programs existed, and if they did, they had a misconception they couldn't access them. Friends or family members might assist with information gathering as well. They might know someone who received home care before, or they may have a career as a health care professional with insider system knowledge. Unfortunately, that doesn't always help. However, attending a support group for family caregivers can also be tremendously helpful.

How to Find Support Groups

The experience of caregiving can be isolating, either because you are occupied caring for your loved one or because you feel guilty about expressing negative thoughts or fears with others. If this is you, then caregiver support groups can be helpful.

There are caregiver support groups that accommodate all kinds of caregivers as well as groups centered on commonalities among certain types of caregivers; for example, disease-specific support groups for caregivers of people with certain conditions like multiple sclerosis, Parkinson's disease, Alzheimer's disease, or a type of cancer. There are also support groups for spouses, for parents of children with complex medical conditions, or young caregivers.

Support groups may be online or in person.

Your health care team may know of some in your area, or you can look them up online or in your local phone book.

Some search terms and strategies to get you started:

- Family caregiver supports
- Caregiver support group
- Support group for caregivers of people with (list the qualifier, disease, or condition here)
- Caregiver association
- AARP (American Association of Retired Persons) or CARP (Canadian Association of Retired Persons)
- Look up the local branch of disease-specific organizations
- Look up state or provincial organizations for caregivers
- Look up these organizations in the government pages of your local phone book, sometimes called the Blue Pages
- Your local health unit or hospital is also a good source. However, don't stop at your first call. In my experience, not all health care professionals or local organizations have the same knowledge when it comes to community resources. Be persistent and ask for help until you find it.

As of the writing of this book there are many online groups for caregivers, so if you have access to a computer and are online you won't be restricted to groups in your area.

There are so many different options when it comes to family caregiver support groups. It is a matter of deciding what will

(*Continued*)

work for you. Many offer one-time information sessions, workshops over a number of days or weeks, drop-in or ongoing peer support groups.

Many groups also offer free newsletters that are full of helpful information and stories if you prefer to take a more passive role while you take some time to think about whether or not a support group is right for you.

Be sure you are investigating support groups for family caregivers, rather than paid caregivers who may be health care aides, assistants, or professionals like nurses, social workers, or others.

Donelle

Donelle was a recently retired pharmacist and the primary caregiver for her husband, who died at home of pancreatic cancer. Donelle had many friends who were also health care professionals, including nurses and physicians. More than a year had passed since her husband's death when she told me her story. She had learned more about services that were available after her husband had died and when she was helping another friend who had home care for end-stage ALS (amyotrophic lateral sclerosis).

She told me she had a lot of support from friends and personal contacts, more so than from home care. I asked her how much paid home care she had coming into her home when her husband was alive.

"Not very much. We never had full shifts, or care every day, and I didn't ever have the impression that I could have, which is sort of interesting when you talk about resources. I thought regular daily care would have helped us more. I had twice a week visits and perhaps

I could have had more. I had overnight personal care aides stay twice a week for about a month or maybe six weeks so I could sleep."

"Could you have had more?"

"Now that I reflect on it, I think I could have had more if I wanted. I started with once a week and then I went to twice a week. Because my husband had every four-hour morphine, that's how it worked out for him. It wasn't long lasting, so somebody had to give it to him and that was me...every four hours. I just needed sleep...I needed to be able to get eight hours sleep, and that's all I needed."

"Did you sleep well when they were here?"

"When they were here I slept in the other room, and I slept fine. I never had the understanding that I could have more qualified people, though."

"Like licensed practical nurses, who they could look after the drip, rather than the health care aides?"

Donelle nodded.

"So, did you get LPNs after a time?"

"I did eventually find out I could have asked for that. But that was long after the fact, and from my friend who had ALS. Then, I understood that I maybe could have had a more qualified person in the home." She shook her head from side to side and chuckled. "But that was long after my husband was gone."

"So even with the midazolam drip, and knowing it had to be checked throughout the night, you weren't offered extra care?"

"I was told there wouldn't be anybody here."

"Was it clysis [an intravenous line just under the skin, continuously administering a medication through the night], is that how they delivered it?"

"Yeah. One of them just told me there would be no one overnight. I know it was an issue. I wanted to be very upfront in asking for the midazolam, that we were not asking for euthanasia...that it's about comfort in the last days of life, however long that may be. And

I think we had an inexperienced case manager, and I told them that up front, that I knew that this was a good way to die."

I knew what she was saying. If people are kept comfortable with medication to help their pain and any anxiety, a death in the home often goes very well. As well, hydration is important for comfort, which is another reason for a clysis line—to provide some fluids. Donelle, with her pharmacy background, knew these things perhaps more so than other family caregivers.

"That's what I wanted for my husband. He was already on Zyprexa and morphine. I had many ways to kill him, right?" She laughed.

"Is that how you were made to feel when you asked for the midazolam, that you wanted to speed things up?"

"In the end, that's kind of how I was made to feel because I understood, for one thing…I mean, I've seen midazolam drips run so I wasn't particularly worried about it running. But I needed some sleep if I was doing the caregiving day and night. I don't know really how to run IV pumps. That's the thing, I think I could be taught how to do that, but I could mix the drug if I needed to."

"Right."

Donelle knew how effective midazolam was for comfort. She thought she could have had support from nurses and when she didn't, she arranged for a few friends to come and stay for the night shifts. When Donelle first had the conversation, it was with an inexperienced case manager who informed Donelle that she would have case managers who were nurses in the house the whole time. She was both excited and impressed as she didn't figure that she would have had that level of support since her husband would likely survive for a few weeks and death wasn't imminent. She just wanted to be sure he was comfortable.

Unfortunately, once Donelle thought she had a plan, the case manager went back to her office and looked into the situation further and was informed by her supervisor that she had misunderstood the limits of home care. Ultimately, a second case manager more knowledgeable and less sympathetic than the first case manager said she could not have the midazolam or overnight nurses.

Donelle laughed as she recalled her incredulity. "She did tell me that some of the problem was that they would think I was asking for euthanasia. Now remember, I had said that in every conversation, 'Let's be perfectly clear, that's not what I'm asking for.'"

"I am quite surprised that was the thinking, from palliative home care."

"Yeah, yeah."

I was shocked that Donelle wasn't offered additional support at the end of her husband's life—either by having care aides in the morning to help her with her husband's morning care or to keep him feeling comfortable so she could do other things with her husband other than provide direct care.

I added, "Even though he didn't want more support, I'm surprised it wasn't offered."

"I may have told them I had everything set up, even though it was with a group of friends, and that's why they didn't offer. I don't know."

"Perhaps as health care professionals, we sometimes make assumptions: 'Because you're a pharmacist, you're in control, you've done it all along, you're private people, you don't need anything' and we jump to the wrong conclusion. It doesn't make it right and it is kind of the easy way to deal with situations that *seem* under control."

"Yeah."

There is a lesson for health professionals here. There is a difference between things *being* under control and *seeming* under control. Most of us like to project that we have got things together.

I added, "Perhaps rather than assuming that you had everything under control they might have asked, 'Is there anything else that I can do?' That may have been more helpful and opened up a different conversation that may have led to better solutions."

"Yes, perhaps. I felt that I had to take charge and set all of that up myself. I knew as long as he was getting transfusions then he would have a little burst of energy while his hemoglobin was high enough. He would be a bit stronger. Then I was okay with the aide twice a week so I could sleep."

I nodded.

"As soon as those transfusions stopped, I knew that within a week to ten days it was going to be bad. I needed somebody in the house all the time when I couldn't be home. Just even to answer the phone. I needed somebody there and so I did work through a friend who organized more friends for me and I said once it gets bad, I would like my nurse friends there. So, I set it up all for myself. I never understood they'd give me maybe a health care aide for nights, but then a health care aide wasn't going to solve my problems. If it was a crisis, it would still be me figuring out what the answer was. It goes back to your comment about resources. So, what they did was done well, but if I had a tip for other caregivers, it's that they don't tell you what you can have."

"That is the piece that was missing for you."

"Yeah. They ask what can we do to help you but that didn't help me because I didn't know what I could ask for."

Unfortunately, this is a strong theme in home care. I heard it in my work all the time. It is one thing to be able to select some things that would help if you knew what was possible. However, it is near impossible to know what to ask when you don't understand the system, how it is organized, and which services are offered. Most family caregivers and home care clients don't understand the different categories of nurses and what they can do, let alone the different support workers like health care aides and what they can and cannot do.

Donelle did know the various skill sets of nurses and health care aides—more so than other family caregivers I've come in contact with—but she still didn't know what was available to her. She felt she should have been told about the availability of health care aides or LPNs, or been told that they didn't do short visits at night. Had she been advised of the options she would have been able to make an informed decision which could have made life easier or more manageable. Because things weren't explicit, she didn't know what to ask for and assumed she was expected to set care in place for herself. So, she did.

She said, "I enlisted the help of one friend—Marliss—to organize the shifts for me and I emailed several of my friends who either offered to help, or I knew would be there for me, and said, 'Please contact Marliss if you think you could provide support to us. You know, I don't wish to put you under any obligation, but if you could provide support to us would you please get in touch with so-and-so.' We had friends stay with us from eight in the morning until eight at night, and one of my nursing friends stayed from eight at night until eight in the morning. In the beginning, I would say to people, 'It's ok, we're doing fine, you don't have to come.' And in the end they came, even if they were only here to answer the phone or to say to people 'It's not a good day to come'—that kind of thing. And then the one half hour I did have to myself was when my husband had a crisis. It was 4 o'clock in the afternoon, and my husband probably passed out. I thought he died. And I had the pager number for my palliative care nurse friend, so I paged her and put 911 at the end of it. She called me right away and was here in fifteen minutes."

"I don't think I could have had that support from home care—and that's missing. That truly is missing, that if somebody's going to be that close to the end of their life at the home, if there's going to be a crisis, somebody has to be able to respond in fifteen minutes. Not in an hour or two."

Caregivers need comprehensive and correct information. This enables them to meaningfully participate in shared decision-making about the best care and supports for them—and ultimately to receive the right help for their loved one. Donelle was a health care professional and obviously very resourceful with a strong network of friends. Not everyone has that.

The home care system fails caregivers by not providing timely and relevant information. Helping caregivers know what questions to ask and knowing what basic services are available would be a starting point. While not knowing what to ask is a barrier to getting better support and care, once a client is assessed and receiving home care, in many cases it is very helpful. Donelle was able to help another friend who was a caregiver get information about services because she had been through the process with her dying husband. It shouldn't be left to chance or "who you know" that determines whether or not caregivers have access to the right information.

Donelle continued. "There wasn't one person who came into the home who wasn't good. They were all good. The biggest gap was not knowing exactly what I could have. I told that to my ALS friend when they had been in health care for a while and recently they started getting palliative care. When they first talked about palliative health care, I said to him, 'You ask for everything you think you want whether or not you think you'll need it. You tell them, I need this, and I need this, and I need this.'"

"In terms of the support they [home care] provide, incredible. But the thing is, they don't tell you what they can offer so caregivers need to be told to ask for everything they need because it's probably there." I agreed. There are some good home care programs. However, it shouldn't be an insider story.

I say it often: home care programs and what services they provide are a best-kept secret. That should not be the case. Providing information that helps caregivers—whether it's from a physician, a home care nurse or another professional in the health care system—ought to be one of the first conversations between a caregiver and their health care provider. An intentional, planned conversation should happen at the first point of contact with the health and social system, or at least early enough that caregivers are set up with basic information to help themselves. This is rarely the case.

Health care providers need to start thinking about information sharing as a significant part of their responsibility to family caregivers and clients. Learning what's out there and being resourceful enough to find out ought to be part of their job. It's ludicrous to think if people knew all that could be available to them then they would further tax home care programs by their demands. That home care is based on assessed need by a case manager is information that ought to be publicly available. Most families do not want a swinging door of service providers. They find it an invasion of their space and their privacy. What they do want is assistance that will make their lives easier and add quality to their lives. Most of all, people want information to make the best choices for their loved ones to have a reasonable quality of life.

CHAPTER SEVEN

Beat the Clock

"I don't want to have to do any more 'have to dos.' I want to do what I want to do. A person who is not a caregiver has no clue. It's always 'have to do,' 'have to do,' 'have to do.' When do I get a chance to do what I would like to do? I realize that I'm distracted, and I have too many things to do. My head spins when I think of all I've got to do and then there's the other thing—what I forgot to do. It's too much sometimes."

—Shirley

It's About Time

TIME PLAYS AN ESSENTIAL ROLE in the lives of care-givers. Not only do they experience a loss of time to do things they once took for granted, but everything they do seems to be constrained by it. Caregivers are aware of time, well—all the time. These constraints refer to the burden of time, the demands of arduous schedules, and the need to complete a treatment or administer medication on time. When things don't go as planned it creates a domino effect: the health care aide is late, meaning the caregiver misses their hair appointment, becomes frustrated, and leaves the house without their grocery list. Returning home for the list, now so short on time, they find themselves speeding while driving, knowing they should slow down, but they can't—they need to be back home in two hours! Things are not only out of sorts for the day, but also for the weeks until they get their hair done.

A caregiver must prioritize activities and carefully consider decisions, like when to run an errand or even when to shower or bathe themselves. Self-care can seem like a luxury for caregivers who struggle to get everything done for their loved one. Whether it's their personal grooming routine, their social life, or even spiritual life, they often find themselves bemoaning the fact that a day only has twenty-four hours. When time is of the essence, caregivers will often sacrifice their own needs and desires in order to be able to meet the needs of the one they are caring for.

Myrna

There was no rhyme or reason to the ups and downs of Dad's condition. It was clear, though, that as his condition progressed, the demands on Mom escalated. Everything she did, every time she went out—to run errands, or get her hair done, or anything at all—it was always in a rush. Every moment was controlled and organized around Dad's needs.

So, it came as no surprise when I was home for a short visit and my Mom told me about getting stopped by the police.

"That bastard of a cop! He was right there at the corner where he always parks in wait. It's been a few years since he stopped me."

I was sitting in the den with Mom and Dad.

"I was tramping on the accelerator," Mom told me. I could imagine! Even our neighbors knew Mom had a lead foot. "I took the turn too quickly. I had to get home. I knew your father would need help going to the bathroom and he'd be starving. The poor bugger was home alone all day. I don't know what came over me, Kimmie." She took a breath and laughed as she leaned into me. "I just thought 'bullshit,' and decided not to stop."

"All the way home, Mom? Really? That's about six miles!"

Trying to ignore the police was crazy, even for her.

"Yes. He never put the siren on so I pretended I didn't see him."

She was already stressed and tired and the incident had tipped her over the edge.

"I pulled in the driveway and the cop pulled in right behind me. I walked toward him and let it rip. I said, 'Do you have nothing better to do than follow me home? I have a disabled husband in the house. Why the hell are you following me like that?' Christ, I was mad. Finally, I took a breath and just stared at him." Then, he said, 'Ma'am, is that your husband standing in the window?' I turned and looked. There was Donnie standing at the kitchen window. The timing, Kimmie. You know he can't stand for more than a minute before needing his wheelchair. Anyway, the cop apologized, then left, reminding me to slow down next time. And of course, when I got back to the house, angrier than hell, Donnie had already sat himself back in his wheelchair."

Dad chuckled. "Yes, it was something." He laughed. By now Mom was laughing too.

"I just know your Dad was thinking, 'You crazy bitch.'"

Time pressure is a symptom of caregiving—the feeling that you are constantly in a rush. It can create illness in the body and the mind. It increases cortisol and becomes a physical stressor on the body as it is in a perpetual state of fight or flight. Further, the stress related to a constant state of rushing and having little time can have a negative effect on your mental health, and can also put you in dangerous situations, especially when driving.

Patricia

Patricia, a former office administrator and a caregiver for her husband Vic, described her morning as a caregiver. "I go downstairs and get the breakfast ready, I take his pills from his blister pack, put them on the placemat, I prepare cereal. I get his juice, mix it with Metamucil, sometimes coffee. I feed the dog. Then I need to think, 'Did I eat?'"

She said getting Vic dressed for the day was an ordeal. "It takes a lot of time. I find him standing with his hands out, talking to himself. He used to shower every day; now, tell him to. Everything takes a long time now. Then, I look down and I'm still in my housecoat."

It's a juggling act for caregivers to get everything done in one day between the "musts," like providing care to their loved ones, and the "shoulds" like doing laundry or vacuuming. When care providers come into their home or carers have to attend outside appointments, everything must be carefully scheduled and pre-arranged. Their loved one's health status and energy levels often dictate the order of events throughout the day. (For instance, if they tend to tire easily by the afternoon, a caregiver might schedule their appointment for the morning or if they are less lucid in the morning, they might save it for midday.) Schedules are further complicated if a Handi-Bus (a van or bus with a wheelchair ramp or other supports) is required for transportation to appointments.

The caregiver might organize the Handi-Bus to come at a certain time so that they can make it to their medical appointment on time. The care provider, who might be coming in to do personal care, needs to be ready at the same time as the Handi-Bus. Everything must be carefully orchestrated. If one thing is off, the whole day can go awry, which can lead to missed appointments that might have taken months to book.

In-home respite care, designed to provide support and relief for caregivers through a support worker, like a health care aide, doesn't always offer the appropriate kind of care to provide relief. It needs to be pre-scheduled and often the caregiver wants to have things done before the respite worker arrives. The respite time scheduled might not be a long enough period for caregivers to complete all of their errands or appointments. Any unplanned events or interruptions can derail an afternoon in an instant, such as traffic or someone running late. When caregivers are already stressed, time pressures can push them over the edge, causing them to make poor decisions, as was the case for Mom with the cop. As for Patricia, she found herself forgetting things so often that she was redoing several tasks in the run of a day.

Although respite is designed to allow for a rest or a break, caregivers often end up taking care of business and errands rather than relaxing or taking the time to do something pleasurable. Most leave their homes when the respite worker arrives because they feel uncomfortable "doing nothing" when the worker is in the home. They also crave some private time that is also difficult to arrange for themselves. Privacy is challenging to maintain not only because there is a worker in the home, but because when a loved one knows an intimate family caregiver is home they often prefer them to do certain tasks, like toileting. So, the caregiver usually runs errands, buys groceries, or attends appointments when respite care is present, but only when they can be confident they'll return home by the time the shift ends.

Carol and Todd

Carol and Todd, who cared for his father Max, were self-described "clock watchers," especially on Wednesdays. Like many caregivers, they used their respite time to run errands. They recalled how long it took them to overcome the pressures attached to getting home every Wednesday by 4:00 PM when their respite worker left.

I asked them if their respite care ever lasted more than four hours.

"No, no it never did," Carol said.

Todd added, "It was advantageous that there were two of us because it allowed one of us to go out while the other stayed with Dad. But still, there are times when you just want to get out together, or need to be out to take care of business."

"For a while," Carol said, "while some of Max's elderly friends were still in good health, some very good friends would come over about three or four o'clock on Wednesdays. They'd come over for a cup of tea and a visit. So, if we ran a little bit late while we were out," she laughed, "there was somebody here. Because sometimes it is really hard to always get back right on time. But, you know, for about a year and a half after Max died, if we went out on a Wednesday, we were always home at 4:00."

"A pattern just gets engrained," Todd laughed.

Penny

Penny told me about the patronizing way some professionals talked to her about taking time for herself. And not just professionals—friends, too.

"They'd use phrases like 'Take care of yourself,' 'Feel good that you are doing all you can,' or 'It will get better tomorrow.' At least, she [the case manager] spared me the lecture on 'Looking after yourself is not being selfish.' I never thought it was selfish to look after my needs. As a caregiver, I simply didn't have the time."

Penny told me she was in a state of overwhelm most days. "So much to do, so little time, so little energy. Most of the time when I am at home, I don't get involved in projects that require concentration because I am always waiting for Demetri's call. I can differentiate his needs from his wants. Usually, when he calls, he needs help right away, so I have to drop whatever I'm doing.

"Besides working part-time, I maintain the equipment, house and yard, shop for groceries, run errands, prepare meals, do laundry, look after the finances, make arrangements for medical appointments, ensure that there are sufficient medications on hand, research new medications and therapies, assist Demetri to and from the commode, clean the commode, liaise with Home Care (AHS), the caregivers' agency, various medical practitioners, pick up books at the library...and the list goes on. Someone who lectures me about taking care of myself has just put another 'TO DO' on my list."

Like others, Penny felt buried under mounting tasks. Some were vital, some mundane, but all were necessary. In devoting so much of her time to looking after her husband, Penny was left with little time, or energy, to do anything for herself. Like many family caregivers, she prioritized Demetri's well-being over her own. Just another example of how burdensome time is for a caregiver.

Lavonne

Lavonne also had little time available to do things she either wanted or needed to for herself. She shared how she had to learn to prioritize— what to say yes to, how much cooking she would do, what kind of meals to make that would allow for leftovers, which appointments she needed to bring her husband to and which could be cancelled, how much house cleaning to do, and which friends to see. She was constantly ranking the importance of certain activities and often had to give up on some entirely.

"I don't have the time that I used to have for myself because I do everything now. The house is messy, but it usually isn't this bad." She laughed. "But I do let it go sometimes."

"It doesn't look too bad to me," I said. "How do you find support for yourself, the things you do just for you, amid such time pressures?"

"Well, when I have respite for Bob, or when he is attending his rehab program, I go to the Parkinson's support group. I also have another support group I like to go to and that's the Al-Anon program. I've been a member for forty-nine years. I can only do my outings when Bob has someone looking after him."

Lavonne also talked about scheduling and the time it required to make it to multiple medical appointments.

"The GP we have now, Dr. Stalker, he's the one thing I'm not happy about," she sighed. "I mean I'm judging here, but it's exactly how I feel. He's in a clinic, close to our home. You can go there seven days a week. You just walk in and that's it. But, if we need a prescription, he won't fax it to the drug store, or call it in. We have to go back to the clinic for another visit and I'm finding that it's a problem. He's probably charging every visit and that's money that shouldn't have to be spent. But he has examined or referred Bob for everything. He checked his lungs, his prostate, his hearing, his breathing. He's found us specialists in everything."

"So, you've been referred to many other doctors?"

"To get all those things, yes. Dr. Stalker books Bob in very well, but then after every specialist visit we have to go back to Dr. Stalker. I'm just tired of all these appointments."

"You certainly have had lots of appointments lately. Is there anything that could have made it easier or better for you?"

"Well, for sure not making us go back for prescriptions to be renewed. I figure that the pharmacist nowadays, with all the computers...it should be easier. That's all."

Lavonne continued talking about how the time commitment to get a prescription renewal is challenging. Not only does it take too much time, but it is difficult to get Bob out the door.

"Bob isn't fast. I have to get him dressed and take him with me."

The whole process takes her at least a half a day with getting Bob ready, getting there, waiting for the prescription, going to the pharmacy with it, waiting for it to be filled, and getting back home. Perhaps if doctors realized the time commitment for seemingly simple tasks, they might be more willing to work with family caregivers to make these things easier.

Curtis

Some family caregivers, like Curtis, are active in the care of their loved ones in hospitals and other parts of the health care system. Not all, but many people living in long-term care facilities, known in some parts of the world as nursing homes, also have a family caregiver providing care, advocating for them, and supporting them. Most typically don't move back home, but some do, as in the case of Curtis' wife, Jane.

Curtis was seventy-four years old when he began caring for his wife. Jane had suffered several strokes and was in and out of acute care and rehabilitation hospitals, as well as long-term care facilities, throughout her recuperation. Curtis grew tired of spending every day, all day at the facility, and decided he'd rather move her back home with home care in place.

The pressures are different when a loved one is in care in a facility, but the time burdens are similar. Over a six-month period, Curtis was at the care home with Jane every day from early morning until after 8:00 PM when Jane was settled for sleep. He said it was almost like a death sentence and he couldn't see either of them getting any enjoyment in life.

There are always constraints on time, even within the space of one's home. While some find the time pressures of dealing with paid care providers coming to their homes daily, getting to multiple appointments on time, and the rush that is inherent in morning routines a challenge, Curtis preferred all of that to feeling trapped inside the long-term care facility for twelve hours a day. For Curtis, caring for Jane at home would enable them to have more quality time together. When they were under the same roof again, Curtis felt there would be more time available for his own interests as well as extra time for chores, for errands, and all of the things he needed to do to keep the house running.

There is never enough time and the way most caregivers cope is to learn to let go of some things. In Curtis' case, when Jane was in the care home he let the house go in terms of necessary but non-urgent cleaning and maintenance. Curtis also wasn't eating as well as he usually did as there were more meals eaten on the run so he could be at the care home with Jane. It's not always easy and many find there is no other option, so they just do what needs to be done. Most find it challenging to come to terms with what they live with daily—a mounting "to-do" list.

CHAPTER EIGHT

Meaningful Conversations

"Friends phone and ask, 'How is Roy?' Nobody ever asks me how I am doing or how I am hanging in. I guess people have to learn on their own what it's really like to be a caregiver, the way I did. But sometimes you just need somebody to say, 'You know, why don't I pick you up for coffee?' They don't really get it that even an hour to just go sit out on the deck and talk to somebody else is a break. He [her husband] could be in here and I could have a friend sit on the deck with me."

—Lavonne

Finding the Right Words

WE ALL KNOW THE STATISTICS: tone accounts for 38% of communication; body language, including facial expression and eye contact, contribute a whopping 55%. The rest, a mere 7%, can be attributed to language. It shouldn't be so hard for health care professionals to communicate with clients and their families. Yet, time and time again, as I listened to caregiver stories and the specifics of the conversations they recalled, I noticed startlingly similar issues. It wasn't *what* was said that was the problem, it was *how* it was said. That is, an inauthenticity of tone and body language trivialized their role and contributions and left them feeling undervalued. I was sometimes dumbfounded as I listened to stories about what health professionals said to caregivers.

It can be difficult to find the right words to share with friends or extended family members in a caregiving role. Their lives have changed, and usually not for the better. Some situations are sad, and some are tragic. Most are difficult. Yet, the isolation that family caregivers experience can be minimized by meaningful conversation with others.

Throughout any crisis that causes isolation—a pandemic, severe weather, a natural disaster—people need connection. Caregiving, especially when there are limited supports, causes isolation, but because the problem isn't always obvious it is easily overlooked. Friends and other family members are often the only connection to the outside world, but often the caregiver does not want to feel as if they are burdening others by reaching out. Social and leisure activities drop off either because of the daily demands of caregiving or exhaustion due to caregiving overtime—both of which affect interaction with others. Having friends reach out, if not in person then by phone, email, or even texts, can help caregivers feel connected. Ongoing connection and maintenance of relationships will support caregivers to open up and share honest accounts of what is happening in their lives. Not only will they then be more likely ask for support, others will likely notice they need help in one area or another and offer or make helpful suggestions.

Little Things Mean a Lot

It's often the simple things that can mean the most. Friends and family who take the time to connect, to ask questions, and who are authentic in their communication provide caregivers with a lifeline—one they're likely to reach for when they need it. Communication that goes beyond the phatic or superficial. Caregivers appreciate friends and family who stay connected, people they know are genuine in their concern. So, when the caregivers respond with, "I'm fine" and you know they aren't, probe further. Ask when it might be a good time to visit; respect that time and actually show up, preferably with coffee and a treat, or something meaningful for the caregiver. Unfortunately, many people don't seem able to get beyond the superficial. They trot out well-worn platitudes such as "one day at a time," "God only gives you what you can handle," or "what doesn't kill you will make you stronger."

People often find it hard to communicate in difficult circumstances. Unsure of what to say, they reach for clichés and bromides which are rarely helpful. These phrases can even be hurtful as they can be mistaken for insincerity and the result is that the caregiver doesn't feel seen or supported.

Family caregivers shared what they found helpful, hurtful, and even meaningless in conversations with others. Penny, Lavonne, Lawrence, and Donelle shared conversations they struggled with when people said things like, "You are taking care of yourself too, aren't you?" They found this statement unhelpful and even hurtful because it felt like the person saying it wasn't genuine. Some of the simplest/smallest gestures they found to be compassionate and authentic were when someone would ask when a good time to call or visit was and then followed through, or they spent time to ask what a day was like and then listened, fully acknowledging the demands on caregiver. Even acknowledging that you can see how hard it must be without feeling the need to fix it or offer unhelpful clichés. Knowing what to say—and how and when to say it—can make all the difference to the family caregiver who is struggling to stay connected to life outside their current role. Genuine listening is good communication and is helpful when you want to reach out to family caregivers with confidence, even when family caregivers may be reluctant to ask for help.

Lavonne

Lavonne, a participant in one of my collage workshops, felt that caregivers were often ignored or dismissed. "Caregivers are put on the back burner at all times," she said. "There's always something else to do, you know?" She was talking about the time pressures caregivers face and where they put their energy. Your to-do list doubles when caring for another and the responsibilities are complex. It's not just the physical tasks, but all the coordinating, organizing, and following up with others, all of which leave little time for anything other than what *needs* to be done. That leaves little room for connecting with friends and family in any meaningful way.

Lavonne reflected on something a friend and fellow caregiver once told her. "My friend's husband had ALS. I remember she told me, 'People phone and ask, 'How is Roy?' and Roy this and Roy that. Nobody ever asks me how I am doing or how I am hanging in.' I guess people have to learn on their own what it's really like to be a caregiver, the way I did."

Every caregiver I spoke to would agree.

"But sometimes you just need somebody to say, 'You know, why don't I pick you up for coffee?' They don't really get it, that even an hour to just go sit out on the deck and talk to somebody else is a break. [My husband] could be in here and I could have a friend and just sit on the deck with me."

"I've heard that from other caregivers," I told Lavonne. "When you are on the deck, then your husband can be in the house and you are still at home with him. It gives you the ability to visit with a friend while still in earshot of your husband."

She said, "Yes, if a friend bothered to even sit for a half hour and listen, sometimes that can do a lot."

People often think they need to make a great effort or grand gesture. Nothing can be further from the truth. It's the simple things that go a long way—like the meaningful phone call that lets someone know you're thinking of them, or the text that asks when might be a good time to drop by for a chat. Coffee and muffins, or a meal if someone is going through a trying time, can mean so much. Food can be especially welcome if the person being cared for eats little to nothing or is on a special diet. The will to cook something delicious or appetizing is likely the last thing on the caregiver's mind, but the gesture on your part will be so meaningful. (Stick to something simple though, which can be heated up later if need be.)

Lawrence

Lawrence is a friend and neighbor who was in a dual caregiving role with both his parents at the same time. We met over fifteen years ago after we moved into an acreage beside his parents. He and I got to know each other better when we realized we were both professors at the same university, albeit different departments. Over the years we got to know each other quite well over monthly coffee dates.

Lawrence's mother, Nellie, had been diagnosed with throat cancer. After eight months of surgeries, chemotherapy, and radiation, doctors concluded nothing was working. Palliation was the only option. While his mother's cancer diagnosis and rapid decline was his main focus, Lawrence's dad, Graham, also had a serious life-limiting health condition. Graham had severe and escalating chronic obstructive lung disease (COPD) and was on an approved waiting list for a double lung transplant. His health status was compromised— he was on continual oxygen—and he easily developed infections that needed aggressive treatment in hospital, often in isolation rooms to protect him from any further germs. After her prognosis, Lawrence's mother lived at home, cared for by family. They did not have outside help. The only form of home care was at the case management level.

The case manager did an assessment for palliative home care and arranged for some medical equipment. During the final month of his wife's life, Graham ended up in the hospital with an infection which required isolation precautions, meaning that visitors needed to gown prior to entering his room. Taking his Mom to visit his Dad was a challenge, given her weakened state, so she didn't get to see him often during that time. I recall one picture where they took her to the hospital as it was Graham's birthday and the whole family was able to have a small celebration in the hospital, complete with gowns and gloves.

You can't make this stuff up. That's what I was thinking while watching Graham and Nellie's tragic reality. Lawrence's caregiving was complex: two parents with concurrent, severe, and catastrophic health situations. While his specific circumstances were unique, there are many caregivers in dual caregiving roles. More and more every day, in fact. But the world doesn't stop when you become a caregiver, and caregivers in high-velocity situations like Lawrence's often feel like they are in a bubble. They feel like they are in a world of their own where the immediacy of day to day is all that matters. They are in an altered reality. Life as they knew it is gone. This new reality is all that matters to them and their family. The world outside—where traffic lights still blink on time, where friends and family still go to work and come home every day, where children still catch the school bus and play sports, where the news still comes on the television at the same time every day—carries on as usual. Not so for family caregivers. There is a new normal, and it is sometimes surreal. Lawrence reflected on that very thing when we spoke.

Lawrence has a twin sister, Sara, who has recently moved back to the area but has a full-time leadership job so is quite busy with her work. Sara has three boys, one of whom is married with two children and a new baby, and although they all play a supportive role, it was Lawrence who took on the role of primary caregiver for his parents. It was serendipitous when I got a text from Lawrence one day last fall as I was getting ready to leave the house for some errands.

"Hi Kim, are you home, by chance?"

"Yes I am. Can I help?"

"Is there any chance you could do a pharmacy run for me...I don't have anyone here to help. I am so sorry to have to ask."

"Don't be at all! I am just going out for an errand so no trouble at all...want me to stop by for details or call me? Please ask for anything anytime!"

"You can just stop in when you're on your way out...that's great! Thank you!"

Caregivers are often apologetic. I knew that. They find it difficult to ask others for help and often feel like they are imposing, despite others offering assistance and support.

It was a grey, miserable day. Wet snow was coming down and the ground wasn't quite frozen. It was easier to drive over than walk across our yards. I entered through the kitchen in the back, figuring that's where my friend would be. I'd been in the home before, but the vibe was different this time. Lawrence's family is friendly and outgoing. We were used to chatting over the fence, usually while calming excitable dogs on both sides. Lawrence's mother was what some might call "larger than life," with lots of friends, lots of talking, and lots of joking. She was skilled in many crafts and hobbies and has a large circle of friends. Not so this time. When I walked into the house, it brought me back to the years in my family home when Mom was caring for Dad, as well as the homes of many of the clients and caregivers I visited as a home care nurse or nurse researcher— going in to do assessments, care, or to interview family caregivers. Lawrence opened the door to greet me with three rambunctious poodles in tow: two of his own and Rex, his parents' dog.

We hugged. It was the first time I'd seen him since his caregiving became all-encompassing and he took a leave from the university, although we remained connected on social media and we texted. "Oh, Lawrence, I am so sorry. For all of you," I said.

"Oh—my—God," he paused. "I didn't expect it to be like this, with the family I mean." He paused again. "People criticize *every-thing*. They think I'm here too much, that I am too involved, that I overshare. We all seem to want to take a different approach. Is it always like this?"

I knew he was asking for my advice, and perhaps some encouragement. "Yes. I see that a lot. Families are complicated and everyone wants to do what's right."

"We are *so* diverse. I didn't expect that. People are totally pissed at me! Les and Colleen didn't think I should have made that post on Facebook. They thought I was totally rude and shutting Mom's friends out."

Lawrence had created a Facebook page dedicated to posting updates about his parents' health. He had tremendous support from friends and family—a few hundred signed up to keep informed and communicate with the family. The post he was referring to said something like, "I am so sorry to have to post this, but we need to severely limit visits to the house. Mom's energy is waning and she's only awake for about four hours, intermittently, each day. Our time with her is limited and Dad will get out of the hospital in a few days, so there's a lot of catching up they want to do. Both parents are immune compromised and they need to be protected from outside pathogens."

Lawrence explained what he meant by these terms so people might understand how fragile their health was. He went on to tell family and friends that they wanted to stay connected, and that Nellie had a phone dedicated to texting. He encouraged people not to call as she couldn't speak and her hearing was also affected due to the removal of her tumor. He gave great assurances that his mother was reading every text. It was a compassionate post, thoughtful, and well written. Several people commented with a great show of support and understanding.

"Personally," I paused, and smiled. "I thought what you wrote was perfect. I doubt many family caregivers have the courage to say what you did. I understood why you did it. I thought you were thoughtful."

I could feel the tension melt off Lawrence as I went on.

"I would be surprised if anyone didn't understand where you were coming from. You need to protect your Mom's energy and the time you guys have with her. I thought you addressed that really well. I am sure it was very difficult to write. And you did let people know how to reach out to you guys on the cell as well. I didn't read into it that you were cutting everyone off."

I was thinking about how difficult it must have been for him to compose that post. I was surprised and almost relieved for him when I read it. I remember my immediate reaction being, *wow, good for them.*

He replied, "It was! I had to do something because people just don't understand and *you* know how many people Mom knows!"

I thought yeah, Nellie always had friends coming and going, working in her studio, people with quilts coming and going for her long-arm sewing machine.. She had a lot of hobbies, and was involved in sewing and quilting groups. She had a collection of antique textiles like quilts, small rugs, and tapestries she had been collecting for years and they were often featured at museums and events and had a circle of friends and colleagues around that as well. People were often coming and going helping to prepare whatever collection would be on display.

"People were also coming here who hadn't seen her in twenty years, or at least in a long time, and they think they are going to have the big catch-up session and reminisce about old times. Then they see her and they can't handle it. They get upset and it's hard on Mom and they don't get it. I had to do *something*. Mom doesn't have the energy and Dad just gets out of the way. "

Although the doctors gave Nellie up to six months to live, I knew it would be only a matter of weeks. Lawrence knew as well, as we had shared a few texts in the days prior.

"You know, most people do understand when they know what is going on. Those that don't get it, well, they are the ones you likely don't need right now. Your mom and dad have a good circle of support."

He said, "I know, that's so true."

I added, "They can call or reach out by text. You said that."

"Yes, for sure I did. I just have to do what is right for us right now."

"Absolutely. It is as hard for people to know what to do and what to say as it is for family caregivers like yourself to recognize what you need and just say it. You did that and it likely gave you some much-needed breathing room. This is not an easy situation. It is demanding, not only doing the caregiving, but also looking after your own energy, and trying to do your best to support the whole family through it. Your parents are both so immunocompromised that extra visitors just aren't safe right now. You did the right thing— and a very brave, necessary thing!"

Get in Touch

Use email or social media to communicate with friends and family.

Setting up a group email, group Facebook page, or even invited Zoom calls can be therapeutic for the caregiver who wants to connect with others. These tools can also be part of an efficient time-saving strategy to keep friends and family informed.

Try setting up a few different groups: one for your most intimate circle that might include only children or immediate

(*Continued*)

family, one for a few of your closest friends, and another for your broader circle. It is up to you to decide what works for you.

Think carefully about how many different groups you want to manage. If you don't feel tech savvy, ask a friend or family member to set this up and manage this with you.

Tips for communicating your situation to others:
- Be honest.
- Be direct.
- Don't apologize for your decisions.
- You have the right to make choices that are best for you and your family.
- Remember that most people understand.
- You might use this for ad hoc postings or you might post a short update once a week. It can be as simple or as extensive as you like.
- The purpose is to make your life easier and to avoid having to tell the same stories repeatedly. If it is something that seems to be causing more work, then it's not likely serving you and you may decide not to do it—this is merely another tool for your tool box of choices to make things easier for you.

Remember, these tools are to help *you*.

- Say only what you want to say.
- Share only what you are comfortable sharing.
- You have a right to decide what you want to make public—even with friends and family—and what you want to keep private.

As Lawrence and I spoke, I noticed a lot of objects that you wouldn't normally see in a kitchen, items that tell you there is way more going on than cooking and family conversations. There were dosettes for medications, big syringes in a drying rack for tube feedings, pill bottles, plastic boxes holding various sorts of things from some dressing supplies, containers, tubing, and medications. Things were labelled and lists were out: stacks of papers with medication schedules; daily notes about Nellie's condition and symptoms; rows of phone numbers for pharmacies, physicians, home care nurses, and hospitals.

Helpful Record Keeping and Information Tracking

It is helpful to have notes and records about care in one place. Tracking sheets for daily activities and medications can keep information close at hand for easy retrieval when communicating with health care professionals and other family members. Here are two templates that may be useful or adapted to suit your specific needs.

Daily notes
To document concerns, activities, questions, unusual problems

Date	Time	Notes

(Continued)

Medication record

To document prescription as well as over-the-counter medications, vitamins, and supplements

Date	Time	Medication	Dose	Result/Comments
March 20, 2020	0900	Tylenol 500 mg	2 tabs	Headache lessened but still there after 30 mins

During our conversation Lawrence showed me the lists of meds and how he had them organized. "Did you do this yourself?" I asked. Everything was organized in the same way that home care or a hospital would keep all medication records. I knew Lawrence was in control. I was impressed with how he had things organized so all family members could stay on track when caring for Nellie.

"I had to," Lawrence said, "there is too much. People think they know what to do and I need to keep telling everyone repeatedly to write things down. If they don't write it down, then I don't know what in hell is going on—when Mom had her last feeding or meds. They think I am over the top on this, too."

I understood what he was saying. Family caregivers have routines and understand what little things work well. They know everything from how their loved one takes their medications to how hot they like their bath water and in what order they like to do their morning routine. Communicating these things to other family members can stave off frustration and discomfort. Written records to communicate with their physician or case managers are also effective as memory is often fallible, particularly in times of stress including intense family caregiving.

All of Lawrence's lists and notes were helpful for communicating with others, including family members who stayed with his mom for a few hours from time to time, and his Dad's cousin, Sharlene, who is helping Graham prepare for his lung transplant. When someone is getting a planned organ transplant there is a tremendous amount of preparation and they need a designated coach who will be with them *all* the time. The coach needs to live with the person, attend all of the appointments, and learn as much as the patient about what needs to be done. They help them with their physical preparation and act as their cheerleader and assistant until the transplant and afterward. In Graham's case, he had seven months of pre-habilitation to get his body, particularly his chest wall, ready to take the new lungs. There is an extensive regime to follow and the patient needs to be as strong as possible for the transplant. Sharlene had been a caregiver to other family members who were dying. She took on the role of Graham's coach and moved in with him and Nellie. Since she was already there during the time Graham was in hospital dealing with an infection, Sharlene stepped in for a few night shifts with Nellie.

Sara also comes and stays as often as she possibly can, as well as some of the grandsons and a few friends. It is complicated managing schedules for all of the things that need to be done and considering all of the skill sets and comfort levels of the other family members. Even though some family members might have nursing or medical knowledge, having things written down that are specific to the care required keeps everyone on the same page. Specific communication records, whether for medications, daily activities and treatments, or even a family communication book that everyone writes notes in can help keep everything in order and is useful for follow up with all health care professionals, from physician visits to home care.

Lawrence looked tired, but he was coping—although, he admitted, barely. He had earlier told me that he felt like he was out of his own body at times and just going through the motions. He said he had to work hard to not let the emotional travesty of what was happening get to him.

"I'm impressed. And agree you need to have things written down so everyone can follow it. There is a lot to manage here."

"They just don't get it. Dad's cousin who is here to help with him, moved in here for the next year and so she does help with Mom some, too. But the problem is that she sometimes thinks she knows better and doesn't bother to write things down when I tell her to. It's a bit of a push–pull. I come in and I don't know where we're at with what. It's just so frustrating."

We both paused in silence for a few moments.

I was thinking about how there are so many different ways people communicate, caregivers included. Some caregivers say little and expect everyone to know what is going on as if by osmosis, simply because they are around and see what the caregiver does. There are those who share everything multiple times—just to be sure they are heard—and assume others will remember the details because they do everything so often and it all seems so obvious. Then there are those, like Lawrence, who don't assume anything and want to be sure everyone knows what exactly is going on, so they write everything down and expect others to, as well. I was thinking that the dynamics in the family might be related to everyone's different communication styles. Rather than appreciating that Lawrence is trying to manage the situation with all of the notes, those that can't be there all the time might be feeling that they are being told what to do. And in some ways they are. The others just don't know the ins and outs of daily caregiving requirements with the same detail that the main family caregiver does.

I asked, "How is Nellie doing?"

"She's sleeping in her room now." He nodded toward her bedroom. "She's managing, but the meds she's on, the morphine, is just killing her mind. She can't think straight, she doesn't recognize words I show her on the tablet. It is completely fogging her brain and she hates that. She finds it hard to communicate with anyone or to find the words she wants. The morphine is doing that, we think."

I could see how that would be a problem. Since Nellie's extensive surgery in April, she had lost the ability to eat and talk. She has a tracheostomy in her throat and a feeding tube going into her stomach. She was now communicating with a tablet to write notes to those around her or to text people rather than phoning them. We don't stop communicating because we can't talk.

When Nellie went into the hospital for her surgery she could speak. When she came out, she had no speech capabilities and would not regain that due to the extensive surgery. They had to adapt to other ways to communicate with her while caring for her. Family members still need to engage and listen to the wishes, desires, needs, and complaints in order to give their loved one the best care. It was another new thing for everyone to learn. For people who have never used much technology, the learning curve can be great, especially while recovering from major surgery and being unwell.

Lawrence continued, "We need to get her on something better that will control her pain but not affect her mind so much. So, the doctor was here this morning and we are going to try her on oxy. I am so grateful you were home. Margaret showed up just after I texted you but she is in Mom's studio. They are trying to get things organized in there and there is just so much to do. She is always here doing stuff and making runs for me." Margaret was a close friend who provided support to Nellie and the family ever since Nellie's diagnosis. Margaret came around to help with day-to-day caregiving. You have to be close to take on that role—and Margaret was.

It's difficult for caregivers to ask for help, especially from neighbors or family and friends who aren't around to see what's happening on a daily or even weekly basis. I was thinking that I knew Lawrence hated to call on me to help, but I was glad that he had and I wanted him to know that.

"Well—and just for the reasons you say—Nellie has a lot of friends that are coming and going. I think the whole Facebook page you set up for updates on Nellie was brilliant. People want to know, but it's too much for any one of you to be on the phone with all the different family and friends, for those who are here and those who are out of town."

He added, "I know, right? Thank God for social media. I don't know what I would do. I can't be on the phone all the time. There is so much of that just with the doctors and hospitals and things I *need* to do."

Just then, a phone rang. I saw he had two cells on the counter in front of him, as well as the home phone. He explained earlier that one was just for meeting Nellie's care needs—the other was for his personal use. This call was the pharmacist confirming the prescription I was to pick up.

I looked around and petted the dogs. The whole time I was there the three poodles were in the kitchen with us, rubbing against me or Lawrence, being petted, needing hugs, and laying around. The family are all animal lovers and there are always dogs around. I was used to that. In fact, between our household, their household, and another neighbor's, there were about eight dogs around at any given time. We had gates installed in our various fences so they could open and the dogs could play together and go back and forth between the yards. I noticed Lawrence taking some notes while he was speaking to the pharmacist. He confirmed that I was coming and who I was.

He hung up, "So, you gathered that was the pharmacist. They will have the meds ready and it will just go on our account so you don't need to pay them at all." He named another medication that I would also get as it was nearly finished as well. He said to one of the dogs, "Rex, go lay down."

"The dogs must know something's not right," I said. "How is Rex doing?"

"Oh God. It's awful. He knows something is up and is so anxious. We have him on anti-anxiety meds." The dog did seem a bit hyper and unsettled. He was different. He kept rubbing against my leg, wanting to be petted. "They are like people, needing reassurance that things are okay, even when they are not."

What to Say When You Feel There is Nothing to Say

We all struggle with what to say, especially when we feel as if there's nothing to say that will make things better. However, speaking from a place of compassion, love, and caring does help. You can acknowledge the situation without offering advice. Ask how someone is doing. Let them know that you genuinely care.

At a loss for words? Start here:

- I can see how hard you are working.
- I see you are doing your best.
- I would love to drop off a meal for you. What do you like or not like?
- How are you?
- What can I do to help? (Suggest things like sit for an afternoon, bring a meal, bring a coffee, run an errand, do the grocery shopping.)
- It is really hard when our loved ones (or friends) are ill.

(Continued)

Be careful with:

- Offering advice.
- Sharing your own stories of whatever they are going through.
- Saying "I know…" (I know how you feel, I know what you are going through), unless you really do know.
- *Shoulds,* such as "What you should do is…"
- *Woulds,* such as "What I would do is…"
- You need to take care of yourself first.
- You are a saint.
- You will get your rewards for this.
- I could never do what you do.
- You are so brave.
- He is so blessed to have you.
- God never gives us more than we can handle.
- "Let me know how I can help" is too vague to be meaningful. See above.

It is okay to just listen.

She continues, "I so appreciate you coming over to do this for me. It's hard to ask people."

I said, "I get it, but please," I paused, "know that I am here for you. I know a lot has transpired while we were away on vacation. I wanted to come over and see your parents after we got back but we also know Nellie can't talk and Graham has been ill off and on with his lung situation, so I didn't want to expose him to any more germs than necessary."

When I talk with caregivers, I try to take my own advice even though it isn't always easy: be authentic, offer to help, be specific, show compassion, and never, never patronize. Caregivers have a sixth sense when it comes to this, a bullshit meter so to speak. Most of us are in the habit of offering ourselves in a generic way. We often say, "If there is anything I can do to help, just let me know." However, being specific with our offers, saying exactly what we can do, is much more helpful than an open offer that puts the burden on family caregivers. Sometimes the offer to caregivers is more meaningful if it is specific. Things like your closeness, both geographically and emotionally, to caregivers and their family, your specific skills—are you a good cook, gardener, or perhaps a health professional who can either help explain some things or offer to do, care or respite?—are consequential and can make a real difference. Perhaps you can help with children if there are any, or pet care and responsibilities like walking or veterinarian or grooming appointments if necessary. Think of your special skills and try and come up with what you think might be helpful—those particular things that you could do and are likely to do better than anyone in their circle.

Authenticity comes through when you are sincere, when you are genuine in what you say and what you offer. It doesn't matter *what* you offer, just mean it and carry through. Offer to do a chore, to sit with the person they are caring for, to run an errand, or to bring over dinner one night. Be sure the caregiver has confidence in what you are saying so they know you are someone they can count on, if indeed they can. If they can't count on you, it's better to not offer anything. It's okay if you can't identify anything specific in a particular moment. But you might want to think of what these things might be prior to your call or visit so you don't draw a blank. Depending on your relationship you might write your phone number and email on a card and note some of the things you could do for them. Trust me, it will be appreciated.

If you can't think of anything specific to offer, saying nothing is even less helpful. Silence is not golden in this instance and saying nothing leaves the impression that you don't care. However, giving of your time can be meaningful to a caregiver as Lavonne shared earlier. Sometimes caregivers cannot realistically leave the home, but they can enjoy a coffee and a visit with a caring and compassionate friend. Listening is an act of compassion and respect. Asking how their loved one is doing—how *they* are doing—can be very helpful. If you have no clue what they're going through, then say that. Something like, "Mary, I can't imagine how hard this is for you, caring for John day in and day out like you do. It must be so hard." Rather than, *"Hang in there. You are doing a great job. You are a hero. You are some kind of angel."* These meaningless platitudes are often said to caregivers. They aren't helpful and come across as uncaring. Calling a caregiver a *hero* or an *angel* are labels, and as common as they are, come across as unflattering. They undercut not just the caregiver's humanity, but the many struggles they face just to get through the day. Avoid saying something like, "Be sure you are taking care of yourself too, Mary." That's the one phrase that regularly upsets caregivers. Although usually unintentional, it comes across as inauthentic and uncaring, especially when spoken as you are saying goodbye.

It is easy to understand how family and friends can sometimes unintentionally use platitudes in conversation if they don't know what else to say. And as well-meaning as some people are, sometimes the language they use seems disingenuous. As for health professionals—that's an entirely different story. Their very roles demand that they have the skills to be compassionate communicators. But that's not always the case. The story Donelle shared with me is all too common.

"There was one case manager in particular, who used to say, 'Be sure you are taking care of yourself too,' with her hand on the door and even if I needed something for myself from her I wouldn't feel comfortable asking. It was like she thought this was something good to say. All it felt like to me was an afterthought."

I believe that in most cases the lack of compassion is unintended. When I hear that a colleague was inauthentic, uncaring, vague, or paternalistic, whether intentionally or not, it makes me sad. I know it's true that not every health professional demonstrates compassion for others. It is horribly unfortunate because even, and perhaps especially, when systems fail and poor policies are prohibiting good care and support, compassionate people who try to help can make all the difference for clients and families.

Parents of some of the sickest children living at home, rather than placed in a care facility—those with complex, life-limiting medical conditions—are in intense caregiving roles. They told me that as long as they felt the nurse or health care aide genuinely cared about their child and obviously *wanted* to look after their child, they were happy. Showing loving kindness was more important than anything else—skills, documentation, or even communication with the parent. It was compassion that made all the difference in their world. Of course, basic competency is a must, but so is benevolent caring. Family caregivers of loved ones of any age say the same; care providers they deemed to be compassionate were their favorites by a long shot. And make no mistake about it: compassion is demonstrated through caring, authentic words and kind non-verbal language. As I often tell students, when you feel you can do little to ease a burden, you can still show compassion. It matters.

Donelle

As a nurse and someone with expertise in case management and home care, I was embarrassed to hear what some health care professionals said to Donelle, the caregiver who was also a pharmacist. There was one case manager in particular, who used to say, "be sure you are taking care of yourself too, Donelle," with her hand on the door knob as she was leaving. This was something that regularly occurred and Donelle said to me, "even if I needed something for myself from her, I wouldn't feel comfortable asking. It was like she thought this was something good to say but I felt like an afterthought."

She said, "I get that there are people who aren't comfortable with dying, but there comes a point where you know can't make your loved one better so you can make them comfortable with whatever means you can. And if that means more morphine, then give them more morphine. You manage the side effects, you know, you do all of these things, and I would do it again for my husband."

She talked about it being a positive experience overall and that her case managers and nurses were mostly compassionate and under-standing. Although she had everything in place in terms of managing his morphine drip, weekends or new people could pose challenges. "We had two case managers who shared our case, and they were good. I don't deny that, but we were with them from May until almost the end of September and that's when we were having the most trouble. We probably saw our own case managers eight times."

I asked, "In total?"

"Yes, about eight times from May through September."

"So, who did you see the other times?"

"Whoever was filling in for them, because there aren't many staff or the ones assigned to us were busy."

I asked, "But when you called and you needed something outside a scheduled visit, you would get whoever was available?"

Donelle clarified, "Yes, some were scheduled visits and if we were running into trouble somebody would come. And so that's when I started to understand why some seemed to be using the one-to-ten pain scale. A new person who isn't familiar with his case can look at his chart and see his numbers [on the pain scale] and see how the patient's changing. I understand the theory behind it."

I asked, "Did you think that got at what was going on? His pain?"

"No, it didn't."

"So, in those times would your husband offer anything else, or be otherwise responsive?"

"No. He'd zone out. I think we had two experiences with palliative care physicians when we were going into the palliative care program. One in July who realized that we were really in trouble, and made personal arrangements to see us, which again was through my friend, my own contacts in the system. We were so lucky in the attention we had. I mean, without asking him, 'on a scale of one to ten.' He asked questions that he could put a number on—probably when he wrote in his notes he put 'depressed' or 'experiencing pain, plus sign, plus sign.' But he didn't have to say, 'On a scale of one to ten, are you depressed?' You know?" She laughed. "He'd have a conversation."

She added, "I understand why you ask that about pain, and I thought as a pharmacist that was a reasonable question: on a scale of one to ten, how's your pain? But in the last week of my husband's life, I certainly thought about that differently. I had a friend whose daughter died of pancreatic cancer very quickly at the age of thirty-three. I remember she was absolutely incensed that a nurse came into the hospital room and said to her daughter who was in obvious pain, 'On a scale of one to ten, what's your pain?', and her daughter said 'ninety-five.' She paused. "As health care professionals, I know we have to try to have objective measures and we practice evidence-based medicine and all those things, but from the other side, as a family caregiver, I see how some of these things drive the patient crazy."

I replied, "What do you think would have made it better for your husband?"

"I think they should ask open-ended questions. You know, maybe at the very beginning, or early on in the disease process when the patient is much better, they could say 'On a scale of one to ten, how are you feeling?' After that I think they should have a conversation, you know, ask 'How would you compare the pain? Is it worse than before? Is it better than before?'"

What Donelle shared is tremendously important to both clients and family members. Health care professionals should be much more knowing and intuitive. They should be able to anticipate, understand more fully, and support families at end of life without frustrating them. When nurses and other health professionals get to know patients and have conversations, they can assess the patient in a more natural manner as they are talking. It is a skill that develops both over time as one gains experience but also as they get to know their patients and spend time with them. It isn't possible when visits are quick.

Donelle continued, "I think it's less about filling out the graph that objectively shows that the patient is changing and more about saying, 'Now, are you feeling anxious about this process?' Or, 'Are you angry? Are you feeling in control? How are you doing right now?' Even start with 'Are you in any pain or discomfort?' Anything to communicate with the patient rather than their own scale."

I replied, "Yes, I hear you say that we're not always client and family centered. There are ways to have open communication with the patient and family and derive the information needed to record things that are important to record. The pain scale doesn't mean so much to the client, even though it is an important part of standardized pain management for health care professionals. Perhaps if visits weren't so short, and nurses took the time to listen to what the patient has to say when they ask, 'How are you feeling right now? How was it when you got up to the bathroom last night? How did you sleep over the past week?' Those questions put context around what we are trying to get at for the patient and a skilled listener can, or should be able to, tell how a patient is feeling and how comfortable or not they are.

We also need to think about what matters to quality of life for the client and their family."

We were thoughtful for a moment. I'm not sure where Donelle's mind went, but I was thinking how we health care providers need more time to spend just talking to patients and families. Not only does talking—and listening—provide comfort, but it can help avert problems before they start. Families might then see that most health care providers do actually care and are able to show compassion. However, in home care, when nurses are scheduled to see five to eight clients in a day and you factor in travel time, their lunch break, and time for documentation and to make any phone calls to coordinate care, that doesn't leave a lot of time for face-to-face client interaction.

When Donelle got up to refill the coffee we had been drinking, I recalled something that I jotted down earlier in our conversation. I flipped through my notebook. "I remember you said something earlier that struck me." I read, "You said you remembered someone—'she really was a shining star when she actually just looked my husband in the eye and had a conversation.'"

"That's right."

I added, "So, all our talk about client-centeredness in health care has huge gaps in it if someone comes across as a shining star and stands out to us because they act in a humane and caring way. Wow!"

Donelle nodded, "Yup."

I continued, "We are reasonably well-trained, highly educated professionals and to me it seems like we're not doing a very good job of talking to our clients."

Donelle continued to nod, "Yeah, I'd agree."

Although I was a researcher and Donelle was a family caregiver, in this moment we were two health care professionals, a nurse and a pharmacist, talking about a growing problem in the system we both worked in. It was definitely a unique interview and I felt fortunate to be able to have this conversation with her.

I asked her, "Why do you think that is? Have you thought more about it since your experience with your husband? Like, do we not want to engage? Do health professionals want to maintain distance?"

Donelle was thoughtful as she said, "The people who gave us the best care were the older nurses, right? I think that's because they grew up in the age before 'one to ten' and they just have more experience. And of course, I know we're not supposed to put our subjective assessments on the patient—we're supposed to have the patient tell us—but, there's a fine line."

She was right. It is important to use the client's own words in how they are feeling, but our observations and assessments provide useful information as we plan the best course of action for a patient. So while a client might rank their pain at a four, a skilled practitioner who knows the patient will observe their body language and facial expression, will look at how much and how often pain medication is used, will monitor how they are moving in bed or throughout their room. Assessment is a complex process and most of it is unobservable to others when done well. Health professionals pick up a tremendous amount of information beyond what the client reports to them.

I agreed. "There is, but I think you've identified a growing problem. I am not sure if it has to do with time, experience, funding, or a festering cultural problem eroding compassion in health care. With the growing number of clients on home care and underfunding, we certainly seem to be losing our ability to be with, and engage with, clients and families in a meaningful way when home visits are not as long as they should be. It is something that concerns me."

"Yes, for sure. I agree."

I said, "So I am wondering, did you ever come out and speak to them about your concerns over their approach? Knowing that's not always easy, either."

Donelle replied, "No, no I didn't. I probably should have. But I honestly think they were doing the best they could. And I guess my objective at that point was serenity. I just wanted things calm and serene and I didn't wish to create a kerfuffle."

I often hear that family caregivers don't want to rock the boat or create a kerfuffle as Donelle says. They worry that if they speak up or get too demanding things will get worse. They need to keep things as smooth as they can be. They settle for "good enough"—even when things aren't actually good enough.

In terms of the health care system, and home care in particular, a culture change is needed. We need to create a culture of collaboration and cooperation where the family caregiver is treated with respect and valued for the resource that they are. Health care professionals need time, which ultimately comes down to how much and in what ways programs are funded so that every home visit is not a rush and time can be taken to listen to family caregivers.

Health care mission and philosophy statements are always talking about "value-driven systems." "Nothing about me without me," they proclaim—meaning clients and family should be involved in all decisions as equal players on their team. Health care systems' vision and values statements often state that their processes are based on mutual respect, compassion, inclusion, partnership, and so on. These words and others like them may be written in policy documents and posted in hospital and health care offices, but they're not always translated into action. The culture of compassion that health care organizations desire, and how they express it, is most often translated to clients and families through the actions of the people who work in the organization. Values of compassion and caring are shared through communication and relationships that develop between the staff and clients and families. Currently the system doesn't value time not spent on tasks, and time for talking and listening are undervalued. There is a gap between the desire for compassionate care and actually providing it. Family caregivers experience that gap first-hand. We need to do better.

Meaningful conversations ease a caregiver's burden. That's only natural. We all feel less alone when we know that others care. Listening is more important than talking. Rather than thinking that we need to give advice, we should pay closer attention to what the family caregiver is really saying. Offer specific help rather than meaningless generalities. Avoid platitudes. Speak with genuine kindness and authenticity.

Health care professionals need to acknowledge the effect of their busyness and words on family caregivers. Being abrupt or too distracted to really pay attention can close doors and come off as uncaring. Unintentional or otherwise, such behavior shuts down the family caregiver, further alienating them—they're less likely to ask for help—and increasing their burden. Family caregivers deserve health care professionals who seek and value their input and who will work with them to make their lives as good as they can be.

Family caregivers themselves can also think about what to say about their own needs before an appointment or a home visit. Sometimes practicing what to say with a family member or friend can help as well as enlisting help from other family members to be present with them when they meet with physicians, care managers, or other health care professionals. Family caregivers deserve to be heard, to be considered a meaningful contributing partner in the care of their loved one. They deserve to both be listened to and heard in all conversations.

CHAPTER NINE

A Sense of Self

Pointing to a yin-yang style of the mandala she had created, she said, *"As I worked on it, I realized that it truly expressed what was happening. That this yin-yang, that used to be a whole, is coming apart. It should have been complementary, but it's splitting apart. One half is how I'm staying in control to get through this situation with my husband, and the other half is me internally falling apart because I like to keep it together on the outside. But inside it falls apart—my brain is falling apart."*

—Donelle

Authentic Feelings

"When do I sleep?"

"It's a marathon."

"Only two hours off a week."

"I'm in a constant state of overwhelm."

L OSING YOURSELF TO THE CARE of another is common among family caregivers. The very nature of the caregiving relationship means that someone else's needs come first. Is it any wonder that feelings of bitterness and isolation come second? My mother, Myrna, talked about the anger and resentment she felt as she tried to keep the "seething bitch" from growing inside her. Donelle talked about her two sides, sharing how she was able to portray a calm persona to the outside world despite the chaos of her inner life.

Caregivers sometimes believe they have to choose which persona to reveal (and to whom), which means they feel pressure to present the face of who they *think* they should be, rather than who they are. It is a psychological strain for caregivers to constantly worry about suppressing their genuine feelings, emotions, and natural reactions. Denying their authentic self then becomes an additional stressor for caregivers in an already difficult situation, which can lead to feelings of alienation and indignation that only get worse over time. It often starts slowly, with the caregivers feeling a gradual distance from their life and themselves. Before you know it these feelings of alienation lead to growing resentment and righteous anger. The caregiver loses the sense of who they are as they internalize these new feelings, which in turn block their usual way of being and force a retreat from both their natural self and from others.

It doesn't have to be that way. Being open about how difficult caregiving is can open the door for strategies to help caregivers maintain their sense of self. Recognition, acknowledgment, and action are necessary to avoid falling into guilt, resentment, and anger. These traps are not only unhelpful, but they can affect a person's mental health and ability to cope. Recognize the early warning signals. Explore where these new feelings are coming from and acknowledge how difficult caregiving is and how the caregiver's own needs seem to be subsumed at every turn. Caregivers often feel guilty tending to their needs, so they put the requirements of the one they are caring for, and others in their family, ahead of their own. Unfortunately, that only perpetuates the traps that can negatively affect their well-being. It's important to make space to talk about negative feelings, and also to do something about them. While others may help through supporting and listening, some of this work is internal and usually starts with the caregiver. If the authentic feelings are negated and covered up, it is difficult for others to notice what is going on.

A Sense of Self

A sense of self is the perception of who we are and what we need to feel whole. It encompasses our beliefs and world view, and also how we regard our purpose in the world. Our sense of self is directly related to our sense of well-being. Without a strong notion of who we are, we'll find it difficult to sustain the mental and emotional capacity to devote to our own personal needs and desires, despite the pressures surrounding us. We all have demands placed on us. Nobody is free from outside expectations. Yet the caregiver is in a unique role in that they are forced to put the needs of someone else before their own. The relentless nature of caregiving and its responsibilities means that people involved in a primary caregiving role often struggle to maintain a sense of self.

It was through observing my mother in the later days of caring for my father, shortly after my maternal grandmother Nanna MacQuarrie died, that I first became aware of the immense personal burden placed on the caregiver. Nanna moved next door to us when I was in Grade Ten. "Ever since I was a kid Mom and Dad needed me," my mother said. "I never had any time to myself. They needed all of us to help with the store. There was never time for us to play with our friends. I went to nursing school after high school and started dating your father. We married soon after I graduated. Then, he was at the beck and call of his father. If they weren't fishing, he was expected to be making traps, fixing something, or building boats. Having time to do what we wanted was unheard of. Then you kids came along, and I was expected to do a lot of the parenting on my own."

I could feel her frustration as she spoke. She felt trapped at times. I would have, too.

She continued, "I remember when you were born, Nanna Polley [my father's mother] called and said they needed me to look after Grant while she went down to the shanty in Caribou with Papa."

Mom was appalled and felt she couldn't do it, but she did it anyway. She rarely complained, and this was one of the few times she told me how she really felt. "You were a fussy baby and I had postpartum depression, likely brought on by no time for myself. Then, I ended up looking out for Mom all those years, and then your father got sick a few years after we moved her down here. I *never* in my life could think about just me and what I wanted. *Never*."

I often thought about how awful it would be to never have time to myself. I empathized with her. We had it pretty easy as kids. Mom and Dad expected us to do household chores, but we also had lots of time to play. Even with Dad having MS, we were encouraged to follow our own dreams. If my parents hadn't made me promise not to let Dad's MS dictate where I chose to build my nursing career, I would have never gone out west. I felt torn when I moved away, like I should have stayed closer to help Mom. Dad told me not to be ridiculous, that I needed to do the work I wanted to do. I was only twenty-one when I started term nursing positions up North, and Dad wasn't so bad in those years. Little did I know my move out to Manitoba would be permanent. It was hard to leave.

Now, thirty-five years later, I recall Mom's words about her needs going unmet when I hear the same refrain from caregivers I meet. They too struggle to maintain a sense of self. I think about my own capacity to be a caregiver when the time comes. I wonder how I'll handle it. And it's not "if," but "when." I think about what

I value—time for pursuits like getting out to a yoga class, sewing, or reading for hours and being lost in my own thoughts; time to get groceries, go to the doctor, dentist, or hair appointments; even going for a drive or on a trip when I feel like it.

The Caregiving Adjustment

Becoming a caregiver can be a slow process that allows time for planning and adjustment. It can also happen overnight. Either way, the caregiver becomes subsumed with caring and adjusting their life to a new way of being. Recently, our friend John had a severe stroke and his wife, Helen, was quickly cast into the caregiving role. Both had been highly engaged in community activities that came to an abrupt halt. Helen became depressed and after a while she recognized that it was because she suddenly stopped everything in her life except caring for John. She slowly reengaged with her weekly golf group, a special group of friends, and that was enough for her to feel a little more like herself. She got both interaction with her friends and some exercise.

My friend Cathy recently moved her mother-in-law into a care home. Her mother-in-law is happy there, but it's so new that Cathy feels she needs to check in on her regularly. She stopped her daily yoga and used that time to see to her mother-in-law, but over time she came to resent not taking her usual yoga class. Although it seems obvious, it wasn't until she was talking with her husband and he pointed out what later seemed obvious—he would drop in every other day on his way home from work, and Cathy would visit her mother-in-law after yoga on the days her husband didn't.

Ruth Anne, a colleague and friend, became the primary caregiver to her parents when they both suddenly became frail. As a result, she had to give up some responsibilities at work. "I just dropped everything," she told me. "Who would have thought it would be like this? Some days I feel like I live with them and just check on my own home from time to time." Ruth Anne's solution wasn't so easy, but she did talk with her supervisor and arranged to have flextime so she could work from home when it was feasible. That solution at least gave her more time to tend to her own needs.

Whether it's work, social, or solitary activity, we all need a sense of agency and control to maintain a sense of who we are. There is not a cookie-cutter solution, and what works for one caregiver is not likely the solution for another. The activities may not be at the same pre-caregiving level, but slowly reestablishing connections with friends and bringing meaningful activities that bring you joy will still have positive effects.

Patricia

I was at Patricia's home for a follow-up interview. "I love quotes, so I looked for those," she said, pointing to her collage she made in the caregivers' workshop. *Success is an inside job*, read one. *Planting seeds to enrich your soul garden*, read another. "I try to water my soul garden," Patricia told me, "but I don't know how many seeds are getting planted there lately."

Many caregivers experience personal health crises during their time as caregivers. While caring for her husband Vic, Patricia was diagnosed with cancer, which helped her see herself more wholly. She told me how stressful it was going to the hospital for twenty-five radiation treatments. In addition to the strain of her own sessions, she found it hard to be in the presence of other patients, many of whom had graver prognoses than she did. "I walked by so many treatment areas with all different people and by the time I got to mine I would be overwhelmed, especially when I saw kids."

This was difficult for Patricia to talk about, but she continued.

"When I went in for my radiation, I would lie there, waiting for it to be over, praying for a cure for cancer. I felt a kinship to all those people."

Praying was an important aspect of Patricia's life, so being able to devote time to prayer, even while she was undergoing treatment, helped ground and refocus her. It reminded her of who she was and what mattered to her. She continued to attend church, either bringing her husband along or arranging respite workers on Sundays on the weeks when he was not well enough to attend. Patricia said she also found strength in little books of short inspirational messages or life lessons like the Chicken Soup series (they even have one focused on family caregiving).

Patricia had such a strong sense of self and knew how to preserve it through the challenges both of caregiving for her husband, who had Parkinson's-related dementia, and her own cancer diagnosis and treatment. She is one of those beautiful souls who is a joy to be around. She emanated a positive energy every time I saw her, despite the hardships she was enduring. I am not sure if her faith in God is what helped her stay centered and positive, but I suspect it was a major part of it.

Spirituality and the Self

Spirituality has been long recognized as a buffer against stress and a viable strategy to help overcome feelings of distress or manage difficult situations. It helps with our attitude and outlook when we recognize the world is bigger than us; it helps us feel more harmonious and positive and can help us focus on what matters. In short, spirituality gives our life context and promotes our thinking about the bigger search for meaning in life. Spirituality and faith can contribute to our sense of self, not only through belief and prayer specifically but also through music, meditation, nature, art, or other activities.

Whether it embodies faith in a deity such as God, Allah, Buddha, or some other religious symbol or figure, a spiritual practice can help us reflect on what is happening, rather than navigating blindly through life. Beyond our search for meaning and connection, spirituality helps us release control and eases some of our burden. Quiet time spent in prayer or mediation gives us time for reflection and gratitude. It promotes mental and emotional health and it expands our social support, particularly when our spiritual practice is connected with a community or group.

Caregivers feel they always have to be doing something. They need to give themselves permission to carve out time and space to be with their own thoughts—time to reflect, pray, meditate, think, appreciate, and even grieve. Maintaining leisure and personal activities can help.

Although it's not always easy for caregivers to make room for themselves, outside interests help caregivers preserve a sense of self in order to become the attentive and loving caregiver they want to be. Many find time for reflection by going for a walk in nature, gardening, sewing, woodworking, cooking, knitting, or accessing some other creative outlet. Activities to promote self-reflection can help family caregivers become more aware of their experience and might prompt them to either take personal action or seek counselling.

The effects of caregiving on caregivers, including how it affects their mental health and sense of self, or loss thereof, needs more attention from those supporting them. Health systems owe this as much attention as we give to other aspects of care. It should also be a focus of education programs for health professionals to ensure that they are better able to support the unique needs of family caregivers.

Whereas spiritual practices connected to a religious practice were long thought of as pathologic by psychiatrists like Jean Charcot and Sigmund Freud, they are now considered an important aspect of people's mental health and well-being. Yet, health care professionals do not necessarily receive sufficient education in this aspect of health, nor is it encultured as a valued aspect of care.

As caregivers adapt to their caregiving role, their sense of self is altered through the process of change, loss, and grief; yet there is little attention or recognition for the change and the grief process they are going through. Although research tells us that it can take as long as two years to move through the grief process, there is little attention paid to the effect of change, loss, and grief in caregiving. By supporting caregivers with their sense of self and their mental health as they move through these cycles of change, it might help them to better cope with their role as a primary caregiver. Otherwise, they may turn on autopilot, losing the desire to meet their own needs over the care for another, which over time can lead to unhealthy behaviors or an inability to cope altogether.

Caregiving takes a toll. While health professionals may acknowledge this, we need to move beyond acknowledgment and acceptance to meaningful interventions, like better education for health care professionals to support caregivers as well as policy changes to address the unique needs of caregivers. As it stands, health care interventions are designed to only address direct client issues; insofar as messaging and policy documents are concerned, they may state that family caregivers are part of the focus of care, when in fact they are not. The result is that family caregivers are typically left to their own devices to a) determine that they might not be faring as well as they could be, b) identify that they actually have needs requiring support, and ultimately c) conclude that it is up to them to find solutions and support to help themselves. Addressing the right of family caregivers to their own mental health and well-being should be a key strategy in any policy that relates to family caregivers.

Lavonne

Lavonne (now in her eighties) and her husband, Bill, lived an active life in Arizona, where they started spending their winters a few years prior to Bill's Parkinson's diagnosis. They recently moved into a condo in an assisted living environment in Edmonton where they can access the support and services they needed. Lavonne shared how her husband's illness affected their sense of life as a couple—and how it also affected her.

"Our social life is gone to the dogs. I think we were overactive for our age, really, until this all hit us, but we were pretty good until a couple of years ago. Since we moved into this condo, we've really slowed down. We still play cards, but we can't travel as much, nor does Bill seem to want to. It bothers me that last week I talked to his psychiatrist about going to South America where our family lives and he said, 'He can go, there's no problem there.' But my husband still refused to go." Lavonne paused.

"He doesn't want to do anything. It seems like he doesn't care if he has friends or not anymore. I keep after him, and say things, like 'Bill, you're happy when somebody calls, why don't you call someone?' Even if he doesn't need his friends and social activities, I do. So, I decided I will just have to do things without him for my own needs."

"I started volunteering more. I need people. Not long ago, I volunteered for the Parkinson's Society all day at the Royal Alex Hospital, so Bill went to lunch with his brother. That was pretty good. But if I don't push him, he won't do anything. I don't have the time that I used to have for myself because I do everything now. I have to make time for me."

Lavonne turned to volunteering to get out and to be around other people. Despite being pressed for time because of her caregiving duties, she prioritizes volunteering because she says that it is the one thing she does for herself.

"I do it for me, but I started a while ago because the company I used to work for donates a thousand dollars to any non-profit organization their employees volunteer at for a year. I don't have money to give them, but I can sure give them my time."

While volunteering helps Lavonne stay busy and maintain her sense of self, she has been heavily impacted by Bill's diagnosis, as has her family.

She gestured to a photograph on the table of three kids between the ages of two and seven. "My grandkids are one of the most important things in my life."

"How many grandkids do you have?

"Five," she smiled. "Three in South America and two in Ontario."

"So, you don't get to see them enough, I bet."

She stopped smiling and her brow furrowed. "Well, we did get to see them quite a bit in the past. We've been to South America eight times to visit our granddaughters. We loved to travel. Last year we had to sell our place in Arizona, and I never thought that would have come so soon as we only had it for two years. We had to sell because the exchange rates on our dollar started to get bad, then health insurance for travelling got so expensive. With health conditions it becomes very expensive to buy medical insurance. Sometimes now I feel trapped."

"As a caregiver, you mean?"

"Yeah, not being able to do what we used to do. It was like losing a huge piece of who we were, who we are. [But] I think if you play with those chains long enough you can wriggle out of them. Or, you can try." She laughed.

In Lavonne's case, she recognized she wasn't happy. She thought about what they, and she alone, liked to do. She recognized that even though her husband no longer felt a need to do some of the things they loved to do together, she still did. She made the decision to do things for herself and to find a way to do them. In her case, it was making time for volunteering, talking with her friends on the phone, and maintaining her social connections. If she wanted to go out, and Bill didn't, then she took it upon herself to arrange for him to spend time with his brother.

Olivia

Olivia, an attractive woman in her seventies, started performing stand-up comedy later in life. Well-spoken and out-spoken, she likely used her stand-up skills to advocate for what she needed.

"I don't want anymore 'have to dos.' It's always 'have to do' this and 'have to do' that. When do I get a chance to do what I want to?"

I asked, "So, who or what supports you as a caregiver? What helps you manage and lets you do some of those things you want to do? I know you mentioned you have your stand-up comedy that you love, and you are trying to keep your relationships with friends. What supports help you be able to do that?"

"Well, I have my son and daughter-in-law. My son has gone to every single appointment. My daughter-in-law's been there for everything, too. They're supportive and our care aides are super. It took a while, but we have good ones now because we hired them directly through self-managed care. We didn't like all the different people and short shifts from home care, so we applied and got the funding ourselves to hire our own. Our current caregivers are like family. They encourage me to go out, they'll do extra for me. I don't have to worry about what they are doing and that helps."

I nodded, understanding the relief that having paid help often offers families. "Can you tell me about some other aspects of caregiving that have affected you?" I asked.

"Well, I find myself sometimes wandering in my thoughts. I told our care aide the other day, 'I think you're going to have two of us to look after.' I said that because I realize that I'm distracted. I just have too many things to do. My head spins when I think of all I've got to do—this, this, this and this and then there's the other thing and then I go, oh I forgot that, and that."

Olivia articulated the time pressures that caregivers experience, not just with the tasks they need to do, but all the balls they need to keep in the air: the planning to be sure everything gets done, and communicating what they need to the right people. It is a lot for anyone, let alone for caregivers who often feel like they are in new territory. They are learning what they need to do as a caregiver, and in many cases, they are taking over household chores and responsibilities previously assumed by their spouse. So, beyond caregiving, they are now doing what used to be the work of two people to manage their home and their life. Despite the benefits of the support she does receive, she adds, "It's still not the same kind of support as being with a husband."

Olivia shook her head. "It's too much sometimes. I recently stood up two people for lunch. I've never done that in my entire life. I was busy on the phone dealing with Canada Revenue about our pension and taxes, because I have got to do everything now, even though my husband did all of that. I was on the phone thinking to myself, *when I hang up I'll have a nice lunch afterward*. Meanwhile, I stood somebody up. I was so upset about it. That's just not me."

"It sounds like it is overwhelming sometimes."

"Yes, it sure is."

I asked Olivia to tell me about the other ways that caregiving has impacted her life.

"I wish more people could understand what dementia is. People don't know what to do so I've been handing out Alzheimer's brochures. We need help, but we also need to still be a part of society, not shunned by society. When my husband is with people, he is so funny and it's a relief for me, too, because I feel we're still normal. I need to be with normal people. My husband and I don't have much conversation anymore."

She was quiet in thought for a moment before continuing. "My life is completely different now. I'm like a widow, yet I still have my husband. It's even worse, though, because he's here. If I was by myself, I could continue to live my life as I like. We used to do things together. We travelled together, we cooked together, we gardened together. We did everything together. Now, I'm by myself and there are people we used to associate with—especially family—that have fallen off our radar, or us theirs. Quite a few of our friends have disappeared, too. They just don't know what to do and I'm trying to let them know what's happening. That's what I'm trying to work on with the brochures from the Alzheimer's Society that I give out. It's not because I want to, it's because I have to, so that things will be better for us as the people around us gain more awareness. It goes back to all these 'have to dos.'"

It's essential for caregivers and the family member or friend they are caring for to feel like they are part of a community. Yet we, as a society, are not doing what needs to be done to allow them to continue to engage. We should be having open conversation with health professionals and policy-makers about the needs of family caregivers and the importance of helping them to stay mentally healthy and supporting them in preserving a healthy sense of self throughout their caregiving. And we should educate both the general public and all those who potentially interact with caregivers, like grocery store clerks and hairdressers, on how to recognize and support family caregivers. This might create a more supportive community overall. We also need to think about structural changes that would make it easy for people to contribute and participate in life outside their homes or a clinic until they no longer want to, rather than because it is impossible.

Olivia found support for her own needs as well as her new role in family caregiving by shifting her stand-up comedy routines to talk about her life, with both compassion and humor. She talked to her health care aides about the changes she was going through and her own needs. Olivia also felt it was important to advocate, so she took it on herself to talk to her support system at the Alzheimer's Society specifically about the needs of family caregivers and how they could better address them—she advocated. She started writing everything down so she wouldn't forget things and to free up headspace for other things. All of these activities helped Olivia continue to be the strong, independent woman she always was and helped her cope better than she would have if she didn't employ them.

Structural Changes

In addition to making changes to social and health policy to support family caregivers, changes to physical, organizational, and operational structures need to be addressed. Examples of structural changes include:

Greater numbers of and larger accessible washrooms for both family caregivers and those being cared for.

Accessible transportation to enable both the family caregiver and the one they are caring for to travel together. As it stands, many accessible transportation organizations will only take the client with special needs, not their caregiver.

Private meeting spaces that accommodate the caregiver and the one they are caring for, both inside buildings and outside where they might be waiting for an appointment or transportation.

Comfortable spaces for family caregivers with access to electrical outlets, USB charging ports, and so on, particularly if they are a family caregiver who still works while caregiving. This would allow them to maintain their work more easily while accompanying their loved one to appointments and programs.

Including family caregivers in signage at clinics for example so they know they are considered in the dyad, or that a designated space with their needs in mind is available to them.

Simple Strategies for Self-Care

Fifteen simple strategies for self-preservation and maintaining a sense of self.

1. Go for a walk, do yoga, tai-chi, or any pleasurable movement activity.
2. Include something natural in your day like walking in nature, exercising your dog, gardening, or tending to your plants.
3. Practice saying, "No." Without the need to justify. If you feel you need to add words, then "No, thank you" or "No, that won't work for me today" are both fine things to say.
4. Practice deeper breathing. Deep breathing to a slow count activates our parasympathetic nervous system and calms the body.
   - Inhale at a slow and steady pace for a count of four and exhale slow and steady for a count of four or five. As you practice, increase to a count of six or eight. As you develop your practice you can add a slight pause at the top of the inhale before exhaling with control for your count. Hold a brief pause at the end of your exhale as you develop better breath control. It might look something like this:
      - Inhale for one-two-three-four-hold.
      - Exhale for one-two-three-four-hold.
   - Repeat and increase your count as you are comfortable. Whatever feels good and natural to you is the right way. Do this a few times a day, or as often as you like for five or twenty minutes.
5. Spend time with people who make you happy or take time to call a friend.

6. Laugh at least once a day. If you can't find anything to chuckle at, keep a book of jokes or humor to read from each day.

7. Pray, meditate, or reflect on something you are grateful for daily. We can all think about and be grateful for many of the things we have in our life, and many of the things we don't.

8. Nurture your hobby of choice. If you have more than one, choose at least one to maintain: reading, sewing, cooking, handiwork, woodwork, exercise. Pick one thing you love to do and refuse to let it go. Even five minutes a day counts.

9. Eat healthy foods. Avoid emotional eating. Replace emotional eating with some deep breathing or something you can do with your hands.

10. Eat one piece of fruit you like each day. It is nourishing for your body and sweet.

11. Take care of your health and maintain your own regular and necessary health care appointments: medical, dental, massage, and so on.

12. Repeat to yourself three times, at least once a day or as often as you need to, "It is okay to take time for me." Or replace this with another permission granting mantra of your choosing.

13. Be sure to do something that brings you pleasure each day.

14. Start a journal: for gratitude, for simple thoughts, or just to note what is happening each day. Getting our thoughts down can be therapeutic but the very act of holding a pen or pencil can also be soothing. It is something we all learned to do as young children.

15. Get adequate rest. I know this one can be challenging for caregivers. If you need to access help, then do so. It is hard to function let alone cope without sufficient rest.

CHAPTER TEN

Mapping Your Way

"Like the Garth Brooks song, 'The Dance'—we had a great dance and I'm glad I took the chance. That's the way I feel. I wouldn't want to have missed it. It's not easy and I certainly don't like it. But he was my husband and always my rock. We had a good life and now it's my turn to be his rock. There are so many good things that we've had in our life and I think we've been really blessed. I think as caregivers sometimes it feels like we are reaching for the impossible. I think there's a hopelessness I feel, too, because no matter what I do he's not going to get better and I guess maybe I feel grief in all of this and then I think, 'what won't kill you will make you stronger.' I think it's better to grow old and be inundated with good memories than to let the caregiving period of our life take all of the good memories away from you. It can happen if you allow it, but I'm not going to let it."

—Patricia

The Land of Vulnerability

FAMILY CAREGIVERS TAKE ON THEIR role by chance, which is why I called this book *The Accidental Caregiver*. The prevailing notion that an accident is not a positive event doesn't leave room for the fact that caregivers may express positive feelings about their ability to provide care; nevertheless, it does speak to the fact that many people are thrust into the unchartered territory of the caregiving relationship without notice.

Family caregivers find themselves creating their own map as they navigate through unchartered territory. It was this sentiment during one of my research studies that led to the creation of a parodic map detailing some of the places caregivers find themselves: the Land of Vulnerability, the Gulf of No Respite, Unknown Channels and Stressful Straits, the Mountains of Neglect, and the County of Contradiction. These were the metaphorical places caregivers found themselves as they learned to self-navigate and redirect their journey with each new phase or transition.

With no reprieve, little support, and a lack of understanding, family caregivers often say they feel like a prisoner locked away from all that used to be normal. They enter into the caregiving role with no prior preparation, no set of instructions, and no knowledge of what comes next. In the beginning, some have confidence. Then, over time—maybe a few days, maybe a week, and for some over several months—they begin to realize they have no idea where they are going and no one can seem to tell them.

The Big Unknown

Have you heard that fable about the frog in boiling water? Place a frog in a pot of boiling water and it will, of course, jump out. But put a frog in a pot of cool water and slowly raise the heat and you get frog soup. Caregiving can be like that. The family caregiver might not notice changes in the one they are caring for, how weary they are getting, or how their own frame of mind or state of health is changing. But changing they are.

The depiction of the caregiver's experience as a journey is universal. In my family's case, there were many times my mother, Myrna, felt that the way forward was a big unknown. I thought that of all people,

I should be able to help my Mom and Dad through their situation. After all, I was a home care nurse and director of a large home care agency. I understood the system. The problem was that I was in a different province 3000 miles away. My mother was also a registered nurse, but that didn't help her navigate her new role as she had been an obstetrical nurse through most of her career and retired early at fifty-seven to look after Dad. One of my sisters and my sister-in-law were also nurses; they could only figure out so much as well. Having many nurses in the family, as well as a supportive physician, helped us navigate better than most. However, it was still far from an easy, straight-forward journey.

There were lots of times Mom felt as if she were stumbling through; that said, our nursing backgrounds made a tremendous difference when it came to hands-on care for Dad. Many of the aides and nurses who came from home care were quite good, but with Mom being a nurse, she was able to demonstrate techniques that were easier and more efficient. So she could manage for Dad and also direct the care aides. No doubt she was paving her own way.

Even the most basic needs such as providing good nutrition caused a major bump in the road. Nutrition affects so much of a person's overall health status. In keeping with the chronic slow progression of MS, Dad went from independence to having his meat cut, to spilling his milk, to using a sippy cup, to wearing a bib, to mashing his vegetables, to using special plates with lips and utensils with hand grips, to my Mom feeding him and giving him sips of whatever he was drinking, to changing his mealtimes so he could be fed before the rest of the family, to giving him only puréed food, and to giving him smaller and smaller portions as his frame shrunk and he started withering away.

When Patricia was talking about Vic's deterioration over time, she recalled that it was often when things took a turn for the worse that she would realize how exhausted she was and they needed to make a change to their routine. It was during one of those times when she realized she needed to place him into long-term care. She realized she couldn't keep problem solving all of the different challenges that arose every day. She was particularly terrified, with Vic's growing dementia, that he would wander off and she would never find him. At the time she didn't know about home alarm systems for wandering clients that can be put on doors or even beds and other furniture. She said she couldn't bear another day of stumbling through with only the hope that she was doing the right thing, never having certainty about anything.

Penny talked to me about all of the research she constantly had to do to keep up with her husband's changing routines, medications, and abilities. She felt that she had to figure everything out on her own, and although it was a gradual learning, one day she thought about all the uncertainty she was living with and it was unsettling. No one knew her husband and his care needs like she did, but there came a point where she said she was doing her best and hoped she wasn't failing him.

My Family

Our family meals went from lots of conversation and laughing to no laughing—only because Dad would laugh and start choking on his food or his saliva, so we had to be mindful. He would also try to talk and start choking. Eventually, all Dad could focus on during his meal was chewing and swallowing. The length of time it took for him to eat a meal increased. In the later years, taking two hours to feed Dad his supper was the norm.

Over the years, Mom accepted some help from home care. It wasn't a lot of time—two hours each morning—but it was help. The care aides home care provided were to shave, bathe, toilet, dress, and feed Dad to get him ready for the day. Gradually, Mom began taking over the feeding because they could no longer feed him without causing him to choke. Most of them either couldn't or didn't give Dad the time to eat that he needed.

One time, I visited home and it was clear that something had to give. Mom was exhausted, and we kids knew she could not sustain herself with the level of care she was giving Dad. Dad was worsening and it was near impossible for Mom to get much food into him.

"Kimmie, I don't know how much longer I can keep this up. I am just choking the poor man! He takes so long to chew that he's falling asleep with food in his mouth. He chokes and chokes. I don't know how much longer we can go on like this. I don't know what I should do. If I don't feed him, he'll die but I *can't* just sit by and watch that."

I knew Mom was distressed about it. I could hear it in her voice and I could see her eyes were tired. It was getting bad.

I asked, "Did you talk to him about it?"

"No. What's the point?"

"Well, he can nod yes or no."

"Yes, I know."

I could tell Mom was nearing the end of her rope. It was getting to the point where it was all too much for both of them. Neither knew how it would end or how much longer it would be before Dad would be put out of his misery. This was killing Mom and Dad was near dead. No one could have done more for my father than my Mom did over the years of his illness. What I witnessed in my Mom's caregiving informed my world view of family caregiving. Family caregivers do whatever it takes for their loved ones—no matter what, regardless of the circumstances or difficulty. They are motivated by a deep-rooted compassion for the one they are caring for. They put the care and the caregiving for the other above their own needs, their own health and well-being—usually because no one else will; perhaps no one else can. And it's why I know caregivers deserve help, support, respite, and attention.

"The next thing is a feeding tube and I don't think he'd want that, Kimmie." Not many people in Dad's condition would have been fed so well. In fact, our family doctor often said, "Myrna, the only reason Donnie is still alive is because of love and the good nutrition you give him." Mom was relentless in the way she cared for Dad.

In listening to Mom talk about her challenges feeding Dad, I knew she couldn't go on as they were any more and neither could Dad. I approached the side of Dad's bed and asked, "Dad, you hear what Mom and I are talking about in the kitchen, right?"

He nodded as best he could, looking straight at me. He could no longer speak, but he certainly wasn't confused, so we included him in our conversations.

"We just need to know what you want Mom to do. We know it's hard on you, choking on every meal. There are things we can do and we need to know what you want."

He nodded. The conversation was hard for all three of us.

"We can go on like this knowing that some days you aren't going to take in enough nutrition or we can place a feeding tube in your stomach."

He mouthed a definite "No," then shook his head.

I nodded and replied, "Okay, then. That's what Mom and I thought you would say."

I could feel my tears coming on. This was definitely the next and final stage. "So here we are," I thought. "After twenty-one years of hoping and misery, he simply isn't going to last without the necessary nutrients." We went back to the kitchen, relieved we had had the conversation and knew a little more about the way forward.

Through the years looking after Dad, there were few, if any, signposts. Getting help at decision points was challenging and finding our way was often trial and error. Information was lacking. Beyond finding information, knowing what options were available in certain situations would have been helpful, as well as understanding how various options might affect the trajectory of Dad's life, or affect Mom as his caregiver. There was no one person to call who could spend time explaining options or assist with decision-making. Some decision points were bigger than others, like Mom having respite care come to the house, while others were less dire, like leaving Dad in his chair for a while longer or giving him his breakfast in bed rather than getting him up early on some days.

Having someone, like a caregiver coach or navigator for care-givers, would have helped. Guidance in seeking the best possible solution, whether it was for out-of-home respite so Mom could get away or selecting the best equipment and supplies for Dad, would have helped Mom. She was left to her own resources when it came to investigating the necessary equipment and supplies. Every time Dad deteriorated or faced a new phase with his MS, we would be confronted with change, new information to absorb, and new deci-sions to make. There never was a formal road map or a coach to help.

Mom was mostly on her own. It was both challenging and frustrating to feel so alone in the role she found herself in. She was hungry for information and guidance, as are many caregivers. Many eventually figure things out while being constantly reminded to put one foot in front of the other, regardless of the circumstances or dif-ficulty. They come to realize, despite exhaustion, that they have no choice but to maintain control. Unfortunately, all too often care-givers feel frustrated, short on time and energy, and even demoral-ized; especially when they get mixed signals, or are deferred, brushed off, or even ignored by members of the medical establishment or social supports that should be there to help them. Over time they eventually learn that *if it is to be it's up to me*. They learn to rely less on others and more on themselves regardless of how uncertain they are or the toll it takes. They learn that putting one foot in front of the other is the only way to continue to progress.

Donelle

Donelle, who cares for her husband, John, commended home care for their services. "In terms of the support they provide—health care aides, nurses, case managers—incredible. But the thing is, they don't tell you what they can offer, so you ask for everything you need. But, it's probably there, if you can find out."

She continued, "I had a friend looking after her mother at home. Home care sent RNs in to watch her mother when she had to be somewhere. It was a short-term, twenty-four-hour period. But I was under the impression that there weren't any RNs who would stay in the home."

I asked, "That might be extraordinary for whatever reason for the client? But I think, too, if people know that there's support, and know where to turn, then even that knowledge could help people cope."

Donelle replied, "Yes. It could. They feel safe. Maybe I didn't try, quite frankly, maybe I didn't ask enough questions. I went where I knew I could get help, from my friends."

I added, "It's the system that sometimes prevents really good people from doing a great job. But therein lies the problem. When there is variation in what health professionals or case managers or social workers openly provide, the family caregiver needs to figure it out on their own."

Donelle added, "Yes, they don't know themselves what to tell the caregiver. And for my husband, being at home was the best possible place for him. It was even better for me, as stressful as it was, because at least if he was in the bedroom, I could be with him here at home surrounded by my own stuff. I could run down for the mail, you know? My kids could drop in and it was nicer to be in my own place rather than sitting in a hospital room."

She paused again, "But there has to be more support. More help to figure things out and help us access what we need without a battle."

Caregivers need to feel that they are supported rather than fought at every turn. Whether it is a caregiver coach, advisor, or someone who can navigate through the myriad of services and resources in the health and social service systems—they need a guide. There are innumerable things caregivers might be able to access if they knew about them. Most don't. Rather they stumble through trying to do what is best with insufficient information and poor to no access to things that could help.

I interviewed over seventy-five caregivers in various research studies and talked and worked with hundreds more throughout my career. However, it was witnessing Mom as Dad's caregiver for twenty-one years that drew me into this field of practice and study, both as a nurse and as a researcher. My mother's journey reinforced that helping caregivers navigate through their caregiving trajectory is not an option. It is a need. The stories and caregivers portrayed in this book elucidate the spectrum of caregiving and the depth of knowledge caregivers need to help them stay on course, without wrong turns and dead ends.

As this book comes to a close, I wish for continued resilience and tenacity for all family caregivers. While all caregivers could bene-fit from more time and information, it is resilience that helps some cope and a few thrive through caregiving. With adequate supports, caregivers might be able to exercise better care and attention to their needs without the guilt and resentment that often accompanies tak-ing time out for self-care. Above all, home care, accurate information about services and resources, and respite care need to be more avail-able, accessible, and helpful.

I wish for a society where family caregiving is valued and rec-ognized as part of the fabric of every community. If you support a caregiver, know a caregiver, or work with caregivers, reach out to them in meaningful ways. Don't let them slip through the cracks. Pay closer attention to caregivers and learn how to communicate better and in meaningful ways. Health care professionals and others who are in a supportive role could demonstrate greater understanding. It is a new normal, not only for the accidental caregiver, but for the whole family, social circle, community, and society. We not only can do better, we need to.

For me, I will continue my work as an advocate and ally of family caregivers—for their role in society and their right to care and supports.

AFTERWORD

I WROTE THIS BOOK BASED ON what others knew and shared with me—what I studied and what I observed, not only with my own family, but also with the thousands of families I worked with over my career as a home care nurse and researcher. To others, I might be considered an expert on intimate family caregiving, but you are never prepared for your own journey. Just as I was completing this manuscript, I, too, became a family caregiver.

My personal caregiving story began on September 18, 2019 when my husband, Bim, was diagnosed with prostate cancer—not the kind that 80% of men might have, but an aggressive type that only a small subset of men experience. September just happens to be prostate health month and according to the Canadian Cancer Society, each September approximately 1,900 families' lives will be forever changed with the words, "You have prostate cancer." Ours certainly was. It threw us both into a whirlwind of unknowing and fear. Often, I wanted to scream.

I thought of all of the things I'd written in this book. Were they true? I thought so. But now, I was the litmus test. Concepts I wrote about crept into my brain. The feelings—anger, fear, confusion; the waiting—for appointments, for the doctor, for lab results, for surgery bookings, for people to get back to you; the anxiety and keeping it at bay; the search for information; accessing the best possible care; communicating effectively with health care professionals through the

myriad of health care sectors to get the care and information we
needed. It all took a lot of energy.

Detection of a higher-than-expected prostate-specific antigen
(PSA) in my husband's blood in the spring of 2019 set in motion
a chain of events that would lead to a prostate cancer diagnosis. It
is recommended that men over fifty—younger if prostate cancer
runs in your family—get an annual PSA check. An increased score is
indicative of prostate issues which can be anything from enlargement
to cancer. In my husband's case, his PSA had been checked annually
since his early forties, given his family history. His father died of
metastatic prostate disease in 1999.

Although an elevated PSA is not always cancer and can also be
indicative of a benign enlargement, it was not the case with us. We
were immediately referred to a urologist and in June we were offered
to take a "wait and see" approach before deciding to get the biopsy.
While this is a reasonable offer, and for many prostate cancers it
poses no risk to the person, neither of us wanted to wait given his
family history.

Bim had the biopsy on August 21 and we were both feeling anxious going for the results on September 18. We were led into the
examining room and then we waited.

I squeezed my husband's hand. "It will be fine, he will be in in a
minute and then we will know what we are dealing with."

He shook his head and looked around as he said, "Don't talk."

He was doing all he could do to stay calm and not jump to conclusions. We sat there together, mostly in silence, for twenty minutes. It felt like twenty hours.

The doctor finally came into the room. He immediately pulled a
chair up close to where we were sitting and said, "I am sorry I don't
have better news."

I could see my husband swallow. I held my breath. My insides
began revolting.

He continued, "It's aggressive."

The doctor waited for us to process this before adding there were options for treatment and he would share those with us. None of this seemed real. I felt like vomiting. My stomach was in knots. I was naïve, assuming this would be as slow moving as a sloth. I felt shaky and jittery—my nervous system went into hypervigilance. I needed grounding and when that word *"aggressive"* entered my head, I recognized signs in my body similar to a panic attack—not that I had ever had one, but I imagined this is what it would feel like. My mouth was dry. I wanted to hold my head in my hands and scream. This wasn't happening to me, to us. But I couldn't, I needed to be strong—as strong as I always was for my husband. This was our journey, but it was his body's fight. I knew I was going to have to be the one to keep him grounded. In order to do that I needed to first keep myself there. I started to breathe deeply—in two, three, four, out two, three, four—telling myself to slow it down as much as I could. I started to relax back into my body and I moved my feet to remind myself the floor was firmly beneath me.

We assumed that Bim would be in the same category as the 80–85% of men with prostate enlargement or cancer—that it would be benign or at least slow growing. But we weren't. All of the questions around what we might do with a prostate cancer diagnosis were stripped away. Aggressive prostate cancer is not run of the mill. The diagnosis was completely unexpected and threw us into a whirlwind of fear (both of us), anxiety (mostly him), study (mostly me), and decision-making (both of us). There was no time to wait, but we had to. Before proceeding, tests were needed to determine the extent of the cancer and whether or not it had spread beyond the prostate. We were dumbfounded, wondering how things could spiral out of control so quickly. This was our Ground Zero.

We left the doctor's office armed with the biopsy report, brochures on treatments, and requisitions for the bone scan and blood work. The receptionist said she sent in the requisition for the MRI and we would be called when they had an appointment. These tests were necessary to determine the extent of the cancer and if there was any spread. We felt shell-shocked and our thoughts were racing as we drove away. We pulled the car over as soon as we found an open spot to use my cell phone to make the appointments. We had already waited long enough to get the bloody diagnosis. We wanted the surgery as soon as possible.

Amazingly, we were able to book the bone scan for the next day. I called the MRI clinic and they did not yet have the requisition but said it would likely be November, a three-month wait, for the first available time. I began ranting and said that wasn't good enough. The clerk said if we paid privately we could get it done in two days. For $1000.00, we could at least get him on the surgery list, so that's what I did.

I immediately called the doctor's receptionist for her to send the MRI requisition to the clinic where we would get the MRI. I told her they would take us Friday, in two days' time, if we paid privately but it also depended on them receiving the requisition right away. Given we had both of these tests booked, we could now book the follow-up with the doctor for the results. For that, the receptionist said there was nothing available for three weeks. I complained and she looked again and noticed a cancellation for the following Wednesday. In less than a week, we would have the results.

Prior to the bone scan, my husband needed to get blood work to ensure his kidney function was healthy enough for the dye that would be used. I negotiated and problem solved for some of the incompetence I encountered from the obviously new staff person on the phone. I actually had to ask for a supervisor in one instance. The dye for the bone scan we were getting had to be on hand and normally that took three days to be delivered to the location we were booked at. The person I was dealing with didn't pay attention to the fact that our appointment was booked at their main lab—the exact location where the dye was stored for all of their sites. If I had not been assertive and knowledgeable about working with the health care system, these tests would not have been booked so quickly. I thought about how often family caregivers have to strategize these kinds of problems in order to get action. I was frustrated, but thankful I knew how to maneuver through the system.

The distraction of coordinating the appointments was a relief from the fear we were experiencing. Our son was only nineteen and every ugly scenario flashed through our heads. But we had work to do so we (I) couldn't let each other stay in that dark place. We talked about our fears and worries openly. We approached this in a similar manner to everything else we do—head on. Our family and a few friends knew about the biopsy and we told them the diagnosis over time. It seemed to take forever to get the results so people stopped asking, knowing we would tell them when we knew. But here's the thing—we had to study, talk with each other, weigh the options, and understand this monster before we could talk to anybody else—especially our son.

My job was to retrieve the science, to study, to decipher my husband's specific biopsy results, and measure that against the options available and the evidence-based recommendations. I learned about the staging and grading of prostate disease—about which I knew nothing prior to our diagnosis. Initially I was aghast. I wondered why I hadn't known any of this. I began my deep dive into understanding prostate cancer. I saw that as my role as my husband's caregiver. Whereas any serious health issue affects a family, prostate cancer is actually recognized as a couple's disease because it affects the partner significantly as well. The numbers related to prostate cancer are staggering enough, but they double if your father had prostate cancer and triple if you also have a brother or an uncle who had the disease.

Our information needs were tremendous. Even though I am a nurse, there was so much to learn about prostate cancer, my husband's particular case, and each of the options for treatment with all of their various risks and benefits. Although we had known there was a high probability that we would be faced with this because my father-in-law had metastatic prostate disease, we had thought annual PSA testing would detect anything early and we would be in a great position to fix it. Unfortunately, this was not the case for us. There was a lot to learn about the disease itself. I quickly learned how little I knew. Only 20% of prostate cancers are aggressive and these are often diagnosed at a later stage. Although Bim's PSA doubled in one year, it was still only six—a relatively low score compared to the extremely high scores some men have. The critical factor was that it had doubled in a short period of time. It was the biopsy that revealed the aggressive type. Cells were present in three of six areas they tested, and he had a Gleason score of seven—the measurement used to describe how prolific the cancer cells are in each of the areas biopsied.

Our urologist knew I was a nurse researcher. At the appointment when we got the actual diagnosis, I told him I was going home to research and I asked for some direction on good internet sites. Even though I had access to the best peer-reviewed literature, I knew there was more bogus information that comes up on internet searches than not. I asked him to recommend the best evidence-based, patient-oriented websites, which he did. He suggested I also avoid random peer-reviewed literature (aka academic journals) as there is so much written that would not be helpful and would just overwhelm me. I listened to him, but I did scan the literature as well and found he was right. I was overwhelmed.

I was thankful I had skills to assess what I was reading. The patient-oriented websites he recommended from reputable organizations were both helpful and enough. I studied my husband's lab work and biopsy results against the excellent descriptors of the disease in the articles to fully understand what we were dealing with in order to be certain of our decision. Those early weeks and months were gut-wrenchingly stressful—for both of us. My husband was happy for me to do the research, synthesize the findings, and present options to him as simply as I could. I couldn't help but think of the family caregivers I'd interviewed, assisted, and written about and how overwhelming they also found information access and processing. I am not exaggerating when I say it was daunting, even with my knowledge and expertise as a researcher. I couldn't help but think we need to do better in this area for family caregivers.

Understanding the nature and extent of his disease helped us rule out treatment options like radiation or seed implantation, sometimes in combination with each other or in addition to surgery. It was clear that surgery was necessary, as our urologist more or less agreed at our prior appointment. However, the patient still must know enough to have input into the decision.

We never doubted the excellent medical care from our urologist. But we were concerned about how accurate he could be about surgery wait times. Even though our urologist felt confident the surgery could be done within three months, he has no control over the many administrative and bureaucratic factors that plague the Canadian health care system. He is assigned surgical slots by an administrative process, then he schedules his own patients according to highest priority. There are only so many slots assigned to each surgeon in any hospital, not accounting for accidents, emergencies, and system or equipment breakdowns. We were open about our concerns and discussed the quality of care we would get here in Canada and how nervous we were about the wait time. Bim asked our doctor about going to the United States—specifically, if it were him in our position, would he wait to get the surgery here? He said yes without hesitation. That was reassuring and we knew he was not placating us.

However, we still weren't confident about the wait times—our doctor could do little about that other than triage us with his own patient surgeries. Right away we began our investigation into going to the United States. This necessitated another round of research and assessment of all the options that were involved. We chose the Mayo in Rochester, Minnesota. My sister had a physician friend who had recently gone through the same surgery there and we had a referral to his urologist. We completed all of the paperwork and were approved. Although we determined that we could afford it, our deliberation was more about the post-op care and the follow up that would be necessary here at home. Even though our physician might have been able to assist us in finding the best clinic, he said he would not keep us on his service. He needed to keep spots open for his own patients, and Bim would no longer be considered one if our physician did not do his surgery. Because our physician assured us we would not be at any further risk to wait, we committed to wait it out and reassess if we were not called within three months. We openly shared our fears about the wait times and he understood. He reassured us that he was fairly confident about the three-month window. The call finally came and the surgery was set for November 29, 2019.

The time from suspicion of disease through to diagnosis and getting the surgery scheduled was mentally draining. Halfway through the waiting period, my husband told me he was starting to feel depressed from the diagnosis and the worry. We followed up with his doctor's registered nurse and she said this was not unusual. She said if it was needed she could speak to the doctor about prescribing an anti-anxiety medication, but in the end we decided that what we needed was respite—even though we didn't call it that—to alleviate the monotony of waiting for the call for surgery. We went to my sister's for a week. It was refreshing to get away and experience a change of pace and scenery and my husband kept busy farming with our brother-in-law. Taking care of our mental health was a necessary step.

Time was a factor for us, but only in terms of fitting in all the appointments for the doctor, lab work, and x-rays. Although I was involved with my husband's appointments and was the one to do all of the research and coordination, he was independent and healthy. Talking about the options for care, synthesizing research and planning for the recovery required time for conversations. The uncertainty with not knowing what the outcome might be required us to talk about the various prognoses we might be dealing with and what changes to our life might be necessary. They were relatively easy conversations. It was harder for me to talk about the research findings and translate them for my husband. The detail I wanted to provide and the detail he felt he needed weren't always in sync.

I didn't experience the intensity of time pressures to the degree that many intimate family caregivers describe, but I did have some. My issues were the challenge focusing on other things while dealing with the diagnosis, sorting through treatment options, and managing all of the appointments and hospitalization. I couldn't easily concentrate on things not related to us as a family in getting through this process of treatment and recovery. What helped was giving up my two volunteer board positions. I took a three-month leave of absence from both boards, one of which was the family caregiver association in my province where I held a leadership role. I did not have the mental tenacity to talk about family caregiving beyond our own experience. I also immediately let my faculty lead—I was teaching a graduate course at the time—know what I was going through and that I might not be able to finish out the term depending on how things progressed. My teaching commitment was the only responsibility I kept and it gave me relief to know that my faculty was aware of what I was going through in case I needed extra support for my course. In all cases, everyone was understanding and supportive. The time and mental capacity I gained from letting go of most other responsibilities was one of the best things I did for both of us during that time. It gave me the space to cope in ways that I needed.

We communicated the diagnosis to our family and friends in stages. At first, we did not share with anyone, including our son, until we knew what we were dealing with. We went through all of the tests, the initial waiting for diagnosis, making our treatment decision, and doing all of the necessary research in private. That approach might not be for everyone, but it is how we deal with difficult situations. The maze of information, the research, and coming to understand the disease was challenging enough on its own. We didn't need opinions or uninformed suggestions. So much of this disease depends on the type and stage—as many cancers do—that it was all we could do to learn about my husband's specific situation. The fact that I am a nurse and a researcher helped immensely with sorting the truth from all of the myths, fiction, and quackery that exists around cancer. But still, we had to process all of it in our own way.

When we were ready, we shared the diagnoses and our decision on a need-to-know basis. First with our son, who was nineteen at the time, and our extended families. Then we shared with our closest friends. Most people were very helpful and even those that weren't intended to be. I did have folks suggest "organic," "natural," alternative, and expensive approaches. I listened carefully, and then researched like hell. I talked to our doctors. The stories around the effects of nutrition, weight, exercise, and rest on cancer are plentiful. While all of these are health-promoting supportive tools, they will NOT cure prostate cancer. I was thankful I understood that without a doubt.

Some of the best supports we got were from our own circles of friends. All of our extended family, whom we are close to, live in other provinces. So while we talk often and are close-knit on both sides, they weren't here. My husband, when he was ready, drew on his friendships, some of whom were friends who also had the disease. Bim was a pilot and still has a close community of pilots at our community airport where he spends time every day. I encouraged him to share as much as he was comfortable with—friends are great supports and spouses cannot be a sole lifeline to each other. I don't find that healthy and it can be a further stressor if support isn't coming from any other source. For me, I shared my experience with one of my yoga groups—a class I attend weekly. All through the time of my husband's diagnosis, treatment, and healing, the women in my class consistently asked about him, about me, and about our son. They expressed deep concern for us and how we were doing. It was both grounding and reassuring knowing that others cared. I felt less alone. Many women were older than I and had gone through a similar experience with their spouses. It isn't that it was my yoga class—it was a community. I had my community and my husband had his with his own group of friends. Each night, we would share who we were talking with, what we were hearing, and what we might expect at the end of each day.

Home care was offered to us immediately post-op upon hospital discharge. My husband had had major surgery, would have a catheter for the first week, and needed pain control and general assistance. I didn't feel we needed the help and thought of all those who do and can't access it. I tried to refuse home care, but my husband wanted to have at least the first visit and I am glad we did. The visiting nurse was helpful and gave us some supplies to have on hand should a catheter blockage occur. Because I am a nurse, she gave me instructions on how to relieve the blockage. She also gave us the after-hours number to call should either of us not be comfortable with me flushing the catheter. Even though we didn't need it, it was reassuring.

Through it all, our own communities were a sense of support. He was experiencing the disease first-hand; I was his caregiver. Both were unique roles. We were experiencing it together, but we were experiencing different things. I encouraged my husband to maintain his routine, his love of flying. I maintained my yoga practice and my teaching. Those things helped each of us maintain our routines and what else was important in our lives. We were about much more than the disease, but it was hard not to focus on it all of the time.

I think for us both it was always there. And, sometimes, it still is. Especially at each six-month mark when his follow-up PSA check comes around. But we can't let it be all-consuming.

Our new normal, following the initial recovery and understanding the 15% chance that it will never recur, means living with weeks of worry and uncertainty around PSA testing time. Practicing resilience in appreciating that this is only one aspect of our lives and knowing that we can overcome anything that comes our way helps our positive outlook. Dealing with the change that comes from any prostate cancer treatment is something we learned to deal with. And even though we suffered a loss and grieve the permanency of the loss, it is easy when we appreciate that we are not dealing with the alternative—metastatic disease or impending death.

My experience of taking on a family caregiving role was fast and furious. I didn't have to "look after" my husband like someone does when they have a debilitating disease like MS—the disease which had necessitated my Mom becoming my Dad's full-time caregiver. My experience was different: it wasn't the relentless day-to-day caregiving that many caregivers like my mother experience. I am keenly aware of that.

This was the way I navigated caregiving and how we navigated the disease and all it brought to our lives. We all bring different skill sets to any situation—different strengths and various ways of dealing with scary situations—and have different relationships. Even with all of my knowledge—for which I am grateful—it was difficult. The things I wrote about in this book were reinforced. Seeking information and understanding the current state of any disease is overwhelming but doing that and arming yourself with the facts is a key factor to coping. If you don't have those skills yourself, find someone to help you. I have those skills, but it was still overwhelming at times. I relied on our doctors for support. Sharing with family and friends and getting support from them was also helpful, but it had to be in ways we were comfortable with, which for us was after we'd worked through things and shared with our son. Others might choose a different approach. There is no map, recipe, or single route through caregiving, but there is help. We stumble into it in accidental ways. As long as we have diseases, relationships, and aging, all of us will experience caregiving in some way. Talking about it and sharing your experience can help others through their journey.

Namaste.

GRATITUDE

BEFORE I ADDRESS ALL THOSE I am grateful for along the way, I dedicated this book to my parents becasue without them I would not have had the courage to tell our family story. Dad, you were taken from us by Primary Progressive Multiple Sclerosis far too soon. Life is not fair, but no one said it was. I wish more than anything, that it was not our reality.

Mom, you set the bar high when it comes to demonstrating what a loving wife and mother does for her family—the personal cost and sacrifice are not lost on me. Watching you also made me highly curious. Often, I did not understand how you did what you did. You prompted the desire to study family caregiving and shed light on what often remains behind closed doors. I hope I can measure up when it's my turn to care—because one thing I know for sure is that I will be, my brother and sisters will be, my friends will all be called to care.

This book was in the making for a number of years. It wouldn't be in existence if it weren't for the many teams in my life over the last few years who helped make it happen, so oodles and oodles of gratitude for everyone who had a hand in supporting me.

First, my PRIDE in Home Care team of research assistants, students, and colleagues at the University of Alberta Faculty of Nursing who jumped in with both feet when I wanted to interview caregivers and use creative, arts-based methods to support them to dig deeper into what mattered.

The multitude of caregivers who willingly and authentically shared their stories. Without you there would be no book. So many caregivers shared their stories over the years—during my time as a community care nurse, as a Director for our large home care company supporting families to experience the care they needed when they needed it, and as a nurse researcher curious about the lived experience of family caregivers. So many stories were shared by my own family, by my friends, and my neighbours who were living through caregiving. You all helped deepen the understanding and illuminate what intimate family caregiving is. You shone a light on the liminal space between what makes a caregiving experience unique and what makes a caregiving experience similar—the place where story resonates.

My team of mentors and teachers over the years who supported my desire to tell this story how I wanted to. The moment I first felt compelled to write this book is imprinted on my mind. It was during a dissertation committee and one of my mentors told me that if I was going to draw a composite character and create one caregiver's experience from several stories that I ought to disclose that to the reader. I implored, moving my hands wildly about, "Therein lies the issue. This IS one person, ONE family. This is happening to ONE caregiver. It is a single family caregiver's story—not a compilation or a combination of a few families, and it has to be told, and more like it have to be told. Because unless you live it, no one knows what the life of a family caregiver is like." That my learned mentors and research committee at the time found it incomprehensible that one family would have experienced the multiple challenges, as well as triumphs, I had described, made me vow to being intimate family caregiving and all of its challenges and triumphs to light. The seed for this book had sprouted so I thank you for questioning me.

My mentors at the University of King's College were instrumental in helping me move from academic writing to tell the stories

I wanted to tell in narrative form. Their instruction, mentorship, and support showed me that writing this would be hard, but also way more fun than the scholarly writing I was used to. To all of my mentors and teachers, and particularly to Lorri Neilsen Glenn and Lori A. May, thank you for your comments, editing, and conversation over my two years at Kings. I could not have completed this manuscript without your thoughtful heart-felt mentorship.

My colleagues—my classmates—with whom I learned to write creative non-fiction, I learned so much from your sharing, critique, and conversation. It was fun to study and play with each of you in Halifax, in Toronto, and in New York.

My editor, Brenda Copeland, I thank you for your keen eye, suggestions, and comments. The year we worked together added value to both my book and my writing life. You helped me find my voice and shape this book into what it is.

My agent, Rob Firing. Thank you for your belief in my work, first by signing me to Transatlantic Speaker's Bureau and later for your belief in my book project and representing me. Your tireless work led to the best place for it.

To Ken Whyte and the team at Sutherland House, thank you for your work in bringing *The Accidental Caregiver* into the world. The whole team was a joy to work with, Ken for seeing the possibilities and place for it, the editorial suggestions from Trilby Kent, the marketing support from Serina Mercier, the cover design by Lena Yang, and the overseeing and getting it done by the managing editor, Shalomi Ranasinghe. I knew it would take a village to make this book happen and I am grateful to be part of yours.

My siblings Shannon, Todd, Tara, spouses and children—you all make my life full. Life would have been so different if Dad didn't have MS, especially given our young ages. I believe our shared grief made us closer. Knowing that we have the love and support of each other is enough. Always.

My friends and family near and far, in particular the special family I married into–Joan, Alex, neices and nephews you have enriched my life and helped me know where my second home will always be. Thank you all for being there through all of my crazy antics and ideas. Thank you for listening and for sharing your own family caregiving stories–its trials and tribulations. None of us are alone in this world and having each of you in my life makes all the difference. I wouldn't want to be on this journey without you especially our dearest friends Sharon and Brad Eyben and Marietta and Dennis Miller. You are our Alberta family and, "Yes, I do sleep!"

My home team, Bim and Matheson. I love you with all of my heart and soul. You are always there for me, wait for me, have patience for me, and support me in whatever I choose to do. I recognize all you do for me and without that, I could never do what I do. You are my life.

GLOSSARY OF TERMS USED IN THE ACCIDENTAL CAREGIVER

Activities of Daily Living (ADLs): Daily personal care tasks required to manage an individual's physical needs, such as toileting, bathing, dressing, eating, and ambulating (moving about). They either do these activities for themselves or have others partially or fully assist them.

Aids to Daily Living Programs: A community resource that offers supplies and equipment for care in the home. The supplies and equipment may be offered for free, on loan, or for a fee. The Alberta Aids to Daily Living Program is one example and is commonly referred to in Alberta as the **AADL program**.

Assisted Living/Supportive Living: A building or group of buildings in a space where varying levels of care are available. People may choose to live in one of these settings before they are ill or infirm with the intent of staying there until death. There are varying levels and varying costs. Services may include meal programs, in-home care or assistance, cleaning, hairstyling, exercise and activity programs, and some even offer long-term care in designated sections.

Care Coordinator: May be similar to the case manager but this person may also be the scheduling person in a home care provider agency.

Care Provider: Someone who is paid for caregiving. They may work for an organization or be paid directly by the family. They are either in a regulated position, such as a nurse or rehabilitation professional, or in a non-regulated position, such as a health care aide.

Case Manager: Assesses and plans care the client will receive in home care. They are often the first point of contact and the family caregivers' main contact for the home care program. In some areas they may be called a care manager, care coordinator, or case coordinator. They may act as the main coordinator for communication with the client, family, care provider agency, physicians, or other community providers.

Client: A person who receives care, therapies, or treatments. This term is often used in home and community care.

Family Caregiver: Family caregivers provide care and support to a loved one who may or may not be receiving care from home care or live in a care facility such as a long-term care home or an assisted living facility. There may be several family caregivers or friends who support an individual but often there is one primary family caregiver.

Fragmented (system): Lack of collaboration or any relationship between departments and agencies.

Health Care Aide/Personal Care Aide/Home Health Aide: A non-regulated care provider that may work directly for the home care program or through a service provider agency that a family hires. Sometimes they work independently rather than through an organization and are hired directly by families. They typically receive eight to sixteen weeks of training in personal care, either through an educational institution or through an employer. There are several terms used for this level of care provider. In this book I use care provider when referring to any paid personnel.

Home Care/Home Health Care: Home care programs may be private, not-for-profit, or government-run organizations. In this book, home care is usually referencing a government home care program that is available in all provinces and territories in Canada. The actual services may be provided directly by the government program or through a private or not-for-profit agency under contract. Clients and families may also purchase services privately or costs may be covered by a third party such as an insurance provider. In the United States, home care may be covered by Medicare or Medicaid but is most often through a private or not-for-profit organization.

Instrumental Activities of Daily Living (IADLs): Necessary activities that require more complex thinking and organizational skills but that do not involve personal care. These include things such as transportation, cooking, shopping, banking, and buying groceries.

Long Distance Caregiver: Family caregiver(s) who do not live in the same geographic region as the client who needs care. They may be the designated contact or caregiver when care is provided by a home care program or in a long-term care home. The **California Daughter Syndrome** is a colloquial term that refers to a family caregiver who is often not directly involved in day-to-day caregiving or care decisions, yet when they come to town they often enter the caregiving scene with a flurry of activity and opinion about the caregiving and needs of their loved one whether or not there is a family caregiver engaged as the primary contact and caregiver.

Long-Term Care Home: A residential facility where care is provided to clients. It may be called a care home, nursing home, continuing care home, or extended care home.

Patient: A person who receives care, therapies, or treatments. Often used in hospital-based care and physician clinics.

Registered Nurse/Licensed Practical Nurse/Registered Psychiatric Nurse: A **nurse** is a regulated professional with two to five years of basic nursing education depending on their title and education program. They are regulated by a licensing body through which the nurse has annual registration and competency requirements in order to receive provincial or state licensure to work in many health care settings.

Respite Care: Care provided to the client but for the benefit of the family caregiver. **In-home respite** is provided by a paid care provider to a client in the home and the family may or may not receive other kinds of home care services. **Out-of-home respite** is provided in a setting other than the home and is designed to give the family caregiver a longer break from caregiving such as a weekend, a few weeks, or perhaps as long as a month. Settings for out-of-home respite may be designated beds in a long-term care home, an assisted living environment, or even in a hospital in some instances.

Siloed (system): a system where people work within closed environments—often completely unaware or ignorant to other parts that are equally closed off, making communication and coordination virtually impossible. Fragmented and siloed systems affect comprehensive service delivery and often lead to inconsistencies or redundancies. Both can have negative impacts on both quality and safety of care for clients and families.

Support Worker, Respite Worker, or Companion Sitter: Typically would not provide any hands-on care but may do light housekeeping, meal prep (but not feeding), and provide companionship and leisure support.